A DOCTOR'S GUIDE TO RECORD KEEPING, UTILIZATION MANAGEMENT, AND REVIEW

DR. GREGG J. FISHER

Cover Design and Illustration
by Stephanie Westphal
717/435-0137

ACKNOWLEDGMENTS

To Tia Fisher

Her patience during my long hours working on this book has been greatly appreciated. Her talent and skills have contributed to the book cover.

To Stephanie Westphal

Her creative skill and talent have contributed to the cover, artwork, and tables in this book. She has helped bring this book to completion.

To Sarah Brady

Her help in editing this book has made this possible.

DEDICATION

To my lord and savior, Jesus Christ.

To my loving wife.

Her help and understanding during my long hours of work on this book have made this possible.

TABLE OF CONTENTS

x

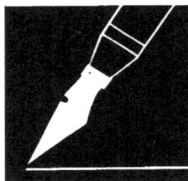

PREFACE

Doctors must be willing to adapt their practices and keep quality records to prevent possible income loss due to inadequate documentation and adverse utilization review decisions. Some insurance carriers require that you submit additional information after a certain number of visits to provide justification for future care. Medicare, for example, has a twelve adjustment limit in each calendar year. Chiropractors must submit additional information in an attempt to gain more treatments. These requirements are not unique to chiropractic. Medical doctors, physical therapists, and other health care providers are coming under closer scrutiny.

Change does not come without "growing pains." Some doctors think that the documentation requirements are too strict and take too much time, whereas others feel that the insurance industry uses the process too much to their advantage. It has come to the point where you must document every procedure well in order to have it deemed medically necessary. As we enter a new century in chiropractic, we must be willing to keep better records for utilization review. Record keeping in chiropractic seems to have lagged behind other health care professions. As a profession, we must be willing to adapt to the changes taking place in health care.

I became involved in utilization review out of necessity for the profession. I have had a small portion of my cases reviewed. Some of these cases were reviewed by reasonable doctors, but some of the cases were reviewed by very unfair reviewers. I started asking myself, how do you get started in peer and utilization review? The answer surprised me. There is no additional training requirement to do peer and utilization review and most reviewers have had little or no training at all. All you have to do is start contacting the companies that "broker" the reviews and market yourself to them. This is how my experience as a peer reviewer started.

What I soon found out really frustrated me. Certain review companies had a reputation for a high denial rate on the cases they reviewed. They would not use a reviewer who is fair or writes a favorable report. I was even asked to change a report because I had approved treatment. I would recommend never working for this kind of unscrupulous company. Not every case I review gets a favorable determination, but my rate of partial or complete denial is very low. You do not have to be performing peer reviews long enough to realize that some chiropractors keep little or no records at all on their patients. Substandard or inadequate documentation is probably the most common reason a case is denied.

What makes a good peer reviewer? In my opinion, a good reviewer must have several attributes. I feel that a reviewing doctor should practice at least three days a week in a clinical setting. This gives the doctor clinical experience and allows them to understand certain nuances that we see in practice. I also believe that a doctor should have been in active practice for at least three to four years before they have enough experience to do a records review. Reviewers should also regularly attend continuing education seminars to stay abreast of recent advances and, most importantly, the reviewer should have good ethical standards.

Reviewers act as referees. They are not advocates for the doctor, the patient, or the insurance carrier. They are impartial observers who must be able to render an opinion without bias to any of the parties involved. Always consider the patient and your profession when making utilization decisions. At one time, only a handful of chiropractors performed independent examinations and peer reviews. Now, hundreds of doctors are performing IMEs and records reviews.

This book provides information necessary to both help defend and document treatment and to serve as a reference for those who wish to perform peer and utilization reviews. Put yourself in the place of the reviewer and critique your own cases. Meet with a couple of your colleagues and review each other's cases. This will help give you a different perspective of what someone else sees when they look at your notes. If you are frustrated with the system, start to perform reviews yourself!

I hope that each person who reads this will benefit from the information contained in each chapter. This book will serve as a reference book for those doctors who want to perform record reviews, but also as a valuable source of information for those doctors who want to avoid and/or win utilization reviews. I would recommend that each doctor attend a post-graduate course in peer/utilization review before performing reviews. There are a few courses taught each year. I have originated and taught two courses on peer/utilization review and independent examination. You may contact Progressive Seminars for future classes on peer/utilization review, independent examination and documentation.

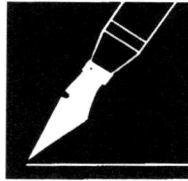

CHAPTER • ONE

INTRODUCTION TO PEER AND UTILIZATION REVIEW

OVERVIEW

WHAT IS PEER REVIEW?

Peer review (S. Haldeman and D. Chapman-Smith, M.D., *Guidelines for Chiropractic Quality Assurance and Practice Parameters*, Gaithersburg, Aspen, 1993): Evaluation by peers or colleagues of the quality, quantity, and efficiency of services ordered by a practitioner.

In some states peer review is done through the state chiropractic board to settle disputes between doctors, patients, and insurance companies. This may also be done prior to determining whether disciplinary action is to take place for a particular reason. In Pennsylvania, peer review is used to describe a records review done under the automobile law while utilization review is used to describe reviews under the Workers' Compensation law.

WHAT IS UTILIZATION REVIEW?

Utilization review: Simply stated, utilization review is the skill of evaluating patient records in order to determine whether the treatment rendered was/is appropriate based on the patient's history, examination, and diagnosis (Fisher, 1997). Utilization review is used more frequently when third party payment issues are involved. This review determines whether the doctor made use of or rendered treatment appropriately. This book contains information necessary to understand the utilization review process and to better document care to avoid adverse utilization review decisions.

As clinicians, we take histories, perform examinations, and utilize ancillary diagnostic tests to arrive at a diagnosis (clinical decision of the patient's problem). Then we formulate an appropriate treatment plan to manage the patients condition. As a reviewer, we will do the opposite. We will look at the treatment rendered and go backwards. We will look at the diagnosis and determine whether or not the history, examination findings, and ancillary diagnostic tests support the diagnosis. Reviewers will then analyze the treatment rendered and see if it is supported by the diagnosis and the patient records.

As you can see, a reviewer must know appropriate history taking, clinical examination, practice protocols, diagnosis, etc. in order to be effective in his/her decisions. Utilization review is not just counting the number of visits or days that the patient has been treated. Utilization review is a skill that not everyone possesses.

WHAT IS OVERUTILIZATION?

Overutilization (Mercy): The provision of more than an appropriate or adequate amount of care in a given case.

WHAT IS UNDERUTILIZATION?

Underutilization: The provision of less than an appropriate or adequate amount of care in a given case.

The treatment could have been effective, but it was provided on a sporadic basis that would not have resulted in a clinical progression of the case. An example would be treating a patient at intervals of several days or weeks during the acute stage of an injury, or at intervals of weeks, when an in-office rehabilitation program was in progress. This would be called underutilization. This may also be due to patient noncompliance.

TYPES OF CARE AND GENERAL DEFINITIONS

Some of these definitions seem very basic but they are quite frequently misunderstood. I once asked a doctor, who finished an in-office rehabilitation program and began again using spinal adjustments and modalities on an asymptomatic patient, why he went from active care back to passive care when the patient was asymptomatic. He responded by saying " I think my care is active." This is why proper understanding of current terminology is important.

The definitions include:

Palliative care: Treatment that is directed at relieving symptoms of exacerbations but results in no net improvement in the patient's stationary condition.

Somatization (Mercy): One of several contemporary terms indicating that the patient's symptoms may be aggravated by or may arise from nonorganic factors.

Active care (Mercy): Modes of treatment/care requiring "active" involvement, participation, and responsibility on the part of the patient. An example of this type of care would be an in-office or home rehabilitation program.

Passive care (Mercy): Application of treatment/care modalities by the care-giver to a patient, who "passively" receives care. Examples of this would include spinal adjustments and adjunctive modalities.

Recurrence (American Medical Association, *Guides to the Evaluation of Permanent Impairment*, 4th ed., AMA, 1993): A recurrence requires no identifiable incident to trigger the medical condition in question; rather, the patient has a resumption of symptoms or signs that can be related to the previously existing medical condition or injury.

Possibility, Probability (AMA Guides): These are terms that refer to the likelihood or chance that an injury or illness was caused or aggravated by a particular factor—"possibility" sometimes is used to imply a likelihood of less than 50%, "probability" sometimes is used to imply a likelihood of greater than 50%.

Therapeutic care: Treatment directed to further reduce symptomatology and improve function through correction of spinal subluxations and treatment of paraspinal tissues.

This should enable a patient to perform most normal activities of daily living without frequent recurrences. Treatment considered necessary to establish a stationary status at Maximum Medical Improvement (MMI).

Rehabilitative care: Directed toward the restoration of optimal strength, flexibility and function of the musculoskeletal system. The goal of this phase is to return the patient to the preclinical status. It includes treatment that relieves exacerbations but there must be continued documented subjective and objective signs of improvement.

INITIAL SCREENING OF A FILE

The first thing that you should do is make sure that you have the right file. You want to make sure that the file you have received is a review to be done on another chiropractor. I am unaware of any state where reviews are not being done by "like providers." In other words, if the doctor under review is a chiropractor he/she will be reviewed by a chiropractor. When the peer review process was implemented in Pennsylvania's automobile law in 1991, this was not the case. Osteopaths were reviewing treatment rendered by chiropractors until a suit was brought by Dr. B. Timothy Harcourt and backed by the Pennsylvania Chiropractic Society. This case was won and preserved the rights of chiropractors to have their treatment reviewed by chiropractors in the state of Pennsylvania.

OTHER INITIAL SCREENING PROCEDURES

1. Look for the mechanism and date of injury/onset. If it is a Workers' Compensation injury you will look for the employer's report of occupational injury or accident report. In auto cases you will look for the police report.

2. Look for dates of any documented exacerbations or re-injuries. Also, look for any new injuries in the same area of complaint as the original injury.

3. Note any prior contributory factors in the history. Determine whether the patient has preexisting condition(s). This may include congenital anomaly, arthritic condition, metabolic condition, etc. This may also include previous injuries in the same area of complaint.

4. Was the patient disabled temporarily? Are they still disabled? These questions may be answered by looking at the HCFA billings. Work modification notes to employers may also give you an idea of what activities the patient is capable of doing.

5. Date of the first and last treatments. If the case has spanned several years or not all of the records were provided, the first date of treatment may be impossible to determine.

6. Total number of visits and charges if this information is available.

7. Organize the file in chronological order.

8. Treatment frequency patterns can be viewed by circling the dates of service on a calendar. This may be impossible if treatment spans several years.

I use a notebook pad when reviewing a file. First, I scan the file and begin to look at frequency patterns, duration of care, cross-discipline examination findings and diagnoses. I am also looking for preexisting conditions and the overall health status of the patient(obesity, metabolic problems, immunosuppression, etc.). Progress reports to insurance carriers, employers, and attorneys will also catch my eye. These may contain valuable conclusions about the current status, prognosis, and ability to return to work in a full-duty or light-duty capacity. I will also note what type of treatments have been tried and get a general idea of the quality of records the treating doctor keeps.

COMPREHENSIVE FILE REVIEW

Once you have looked at the file briefly, you will more closely scrutinize the records in the following manner:

1. *The diagnostic impression is compared with the documentation to see if there is correlation between the examination findings and the diagnosis.* Complicating factors are also taken into consideration. Does the documentation and examination findings support the current diagnosis?

2. *Analyze the subjective complaints, objective findings, mechanism of injury, lab findings, ancillary diagnostic tests including x-rays, cross-discipline examination findings and the treatment plan.* Ensure that there is correlation between the patient history, mechanism of injury, examination findings and the diagnosis.

3. *Review the treatment plan.* What treatment has been rendered or proposed? What is the frequency and length of treatment? Has the treatment plan been modified in response to the patient's progress or lack thereof?

4. *Does the documentation support the care rendered?* Have there been periodic examinations performed to evaluate the efficacy of the treatment and to modify treatment accordingly? Does treatment frequency and modality utilization decrease to correspond with patient progress.

5. *You may be provided records from several different professions and specialties to review.* If the case has spanned several years, the patient may have had several courses of treatment including physical therapy, chiropractic, drugs, pain management, and surgery to name a few. When reviewing records from a specialist you will focus in on the examination findings and diagnosis. You will also pay close attention to the ancillary diagnostic testing and the results of these tests. Does the examination findings from other providers correlate with the treating doctor's records? If not, how do the examination findings differ?

Key findings would include a prior surgery in the area of complaint and failure of the patient to respond to other forms of treatment. Has previous chiropractic care been performed? If not, is a trial of care appropriate based upon the history and examination? If chiropractic care has not been performed, and there is a clinical course with no significant gaps in treatment, then a trial of care would almost always be reasonable. If there was a previous course of chiropractic care, the treating doctor must document a different approach to treatment so he/she does not duplicate a pervious treatment. A mechanism of injury supporting a diagnosable musculoskeletal complaint with a supporting history and examination is typically sufficient to justify a trial of chiropractic care.

WHAT IS A DIAGNOSIS?

Diagnosis (Mercy): A decision regarding the nature of the patient's complaint; the art or act of identifying a disease or condition from its signs and symptoms.

Clinical impression: The clinical impression is a working diagnosis of the patient's case. The chiropractic clinical impression is used to establish the basis and appropriateness for rendering chiropractic care. This is the statement which explains the chief complaint and parameters of the present illness, to include the etiologic factors in standard diagnostic terminology in order to support the rationale for rendering chiropractic care. The clinical impression also aids in determining whether a consultation with another health care provider is indicated before chiropractic treatment is rendered or concurrent with chiropractic care. The clinical impression may be subject to modification as the patient's health status changes.

CONTENT OF THE CLINICAL IMPRESSION

1. *Time frame of condition:* Acute, subacute, chronic, acute exacerbation of a chronic condition.

2. *Mode of onset or mechanism of injury:* Hyperflexion/hyperextension, lifting strain, overuse strain, cumulative trauma disorder, repetitive strain are examples.

3. *Region of involvement:* Regions include cervical, cervicothoracic, thoracic, thoracolumbar, lumbar, lumbosacral, sacroiliac and others. Severity of the problem is graded using negligible, mild-slight, moderate, or severe-marked.

4. *The tissue that is primarily involved and identification of the vertebral subluxation complex:* Chiropractic analysis will reveal the neuromuscular dysfunction. Examples include vertebral subluxation, joint dysfunction, intervertebral disc syndrome, radiculopathy, neuropathy, myelopathy, etc.

5. *Complicating factors including metabolic conditions, obesity, and depression:* Also, include other complicating factors such as degenerative disc disease, degenerative joint disease, congenital anomalies, spondylolisthesis, and continuation of overuse stress or strain.

6. *Organic or somatic complaints occurring at the same time, but may be a consequence (attendant) of the primary condition or conditions that may have no direct*

relationship (concurrent): An example of a concurrent complaint would be one with a extraspinal joint.

A written diagnosis is only found in a small percentages of the cases that I review. It is important that the treating doctor not only formulate an impression about the case but write it in the patient's file. The complexity and length of the diagnosis will be determined by the complexity of the case history, examination, and complicating factors. If you need to practice writing a diagnosis, then practice! A diagnosis is necessary to formulate a treatment plan for each patient and to communicate a patient's condition to employers, insurers, lawyers, and other health care professionals. If you want to refer for diagnostic testing, the facility will most likely want to know your diagnosis or clinical impression and your rationale for the tests.

ANALYSIS OF A DIAGNOSTIC IMPRESSION

First determine the primary diagnosis for the patient. Many times there is no written diagnosis in the medical file so the reviewing doctor will need to look at the HCFA billings to find the diagnosis. Then you will factor in the associated conditions and complicating factors to arrive at an approximate treatment time. This is not an exact treatment duration but it will give you a reasonable estimate. The estimated treatment duration that you arrived at by analyzing the diagnosis will be influenced by additional injuries, documented exacerbations and reinjuries, and the patient's response to the treatment provided. Don't be swayed by an embellished diagnosis. The longest diagnosis does not win a prize nor should it influence your decisions.

EXAMPLES OF PROPER CLINICAL IMPRESSIONS

Acute traumatic acceleration/deceleration injuries to the cervicothoracic soft tissues with attendant spasm of the affected musculature complicated by degenerative disc disease of C5/6.

Acute lifting strain of the lumbar spine with attendant spasm complicated by obesity and diabetes mellitus.

Chronic overuse strain of the right upper extremity with attendant myofascial pain patterns of the right upper trapezius.

Acute overuse lifting strain of the lumbar spine with attendant spasm of the lumbar spine paraspinal musculature complicated by a grade 1 spondylolisthesis at L5.

EXAMPLES OF CLINICAL IMPRESSIONS FROM ACTUAL CASES

"Lumbar sprain/strain, lumbar radiculopathy, muscle spasm."

"Chronic myofascial dysfunction to the right leg, post-laminectomy syndrome, and epidural fibrosis L3-4."

"Cervical disc displacement, cervical neuritis with pain radiating to the right upper extremity."

"Grade II sprain/strain of the thoracic and lumbar spines with suspected disc herniation."

"Post-traumatic acute lumbosacral sprain/strain."

"Acute traumatic hyperextension/hyperflexion sprain/strain injuries of the cervicothoracic paraspinal musculature with attendant spasm complicated by degenerative disc disease of C5/6 and C6/7 and diabetes mellitus."

"Chronic cervicothoracic sprain."

"Acute traumatic cervical acceleration/deceleration injuries with associated spasm of cervicothoracic paraspinal musculature."

"Complication of two crushed backbones."

"Post-traumatic bilateral cervical brachial radiculitis, post-traumatic bilateral lumbosacral radiculitis, rule out radiculopathy, post-traumatic severe grade II cervical myoligamentous sprain-strain with associated myospasm, myofascial tearing, and myofascitis, post-traumatic severe grade II lumbosacral and bilateral sacroiliac myoligamentous sprain-strain with associated myospasm, myofascial tearing, and myofascitis, post-traumatic cervical, thoracic, and lumbosacral and sacroiliac subluxation-fixation complexes complicating this patient's spinal injuries, post-traumatic right shoulder girdle sprain-strain, post-traumatic right wrist contusion, post-traumatic cervical and lumbosacral instability confirmed by surface EMG testing."

WHAT IS A DIFFERENTIAL DIAGNOSIS?

Differential Diagnosis: Determining which condition a patient is suffering from by comparing clinical characteristics and findings of several conditions.

WHAT CHARACTERISTICS WOULD INDICATE A NON-GOAL ORIENTED TREATMENT PLAN?

1. Treatment has not been switched from a passive mode of treatment to an active mode as the patient improves.

2. The number of adjunctive modalities used on each date of service is not decreased.

3. The patient experiences frequent exacerbation's that result in limitation of activities of daily living.

4. The patient experiences no significant improvement in his/her pain or the pain is only slightly diminished for a short period of time following the treatment. This would apply after several months of treatment has been rendered.

5. The objective findings remain unchanged.

6. Treatment frequency is sporadic and would not result in a clinical progression (while in a therapeutic phase of care). This is actually underutilization. In other words, the treatment used has not been rendered on a frequent enough basis or an inadequate amount has been used. The treatment frequency could be sporadic with several days or weeks between dates of service. Treatment such as this would not result in a clinical progression or serve as a therapeutic benefit. Noncompliance on the patient's part could also lead to a "non-goal oriented" treatment program.

Remember, the treating doctor may have a sufficient rationale for intervals between visits. A home based exercise program would be an example. The treating doctor may monitor the patient at an interval of a few weeks to see if the patient is compliant and tolerating the exercises. The doctor may also be using a conditional release or a trial of withdrawal of treatment.

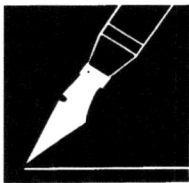

CHAPTER • TWO

MAXIMUM IMPROVEMENT/MAINTENANCE CARE/ SUPPORTIVE CARE

The information in this chapter is very important in today's third party payment system. Some insurance companies may have a provision in their policies for supportive care but not for maintenance care. This is the case in Pennsylvania's Workers' Compensation law.

It is important to know the different characteristics of both so that you can document your treatment accordingly. Have you been told your bill was being denied because your patient's policy did not cover maintenance care? If not, you are definitely in the minority. This is sometimes a common denial tactic on the part of the insurance carrier. Reviewers are sometimes asked to give an opinion as to whether treatment is supportive care or considered maintenance care. This chapter will show you the differences in both of these terms to allow you to better document your treatment. This chapter will also help you understand maximum improvement and how you determine maximum improvement.

WHAT IS MAXIMUM IMPROVEMENT?

Maximum improvement (Mercy): A return to pre-injury status or a plateau point where the patient fails to improve beyond a certain level of symptomatology or disability. End point of care unless there is documented evidence of a permanent injury.

The important point in this definition is a return to a pre-injury status and the end point of care unless there is ***documented evidence*** of a permanent injury. This does not necessarily mean that the patient may not need further treatment, but this means that the patient has reached a plateau where no further regularly scheduled treatment would result in a clinical progression. Some insurance coverages are only responsible for treatment to the point of MMI/MCI, so the declaration of a patient at maximum improvement may have an influence on who pays future medical bills.

HOW DO YOU DETERMINE MAXIMUM IMPROVEMENT?

Determining maximum improvement is sometimes asked during a review. But how can one accurately determine MMI (Maximum Medical Improvement)/MCI (Maximum Chiropractic Improvement) based solely on a records review? The answer to that is very easy. It is sometimes difficult to determine maximum improvement based solely on a records review, but we will cover some areas to key in on:

1. You will first look at the subjective and objective findings and analyze them. The doctor should have done progress examinations at least monthly to evaluate the patient. Look at the examination findings and compare to the previous month's examination findings to see if there continues to be significant improvement or the findings are remaining static. For subjective improvement look at the history but also any outcome assessment forms that were used.

2. Factor in a reasonable healing time estimate with any documented exacerbations and complicating factors.

3. Has the length of time between visits increased? Does a gap in treatment of two, three, or four weeks result in no clinical deterioration? In other words, if the patient does not get worse with two, three, or four weeks between visits, they may be reaching or are at maximum improvement. Remember, the doctor may have a sufficient rationale for monitoring the patient at a two, three, or four week interval. (Monitoring a home-based exercise program for example)

4. Did the patient have any pre-existing conditions? If so, is the patient at their pre-accident condition even though they might have continued symptomatology?

Knowing when a patient has reached maximum improvement is very important. As you will see, maximum improvement is a part of the definitions for both maintenance and supportive care. How could you be performing maintenance or supportive care if you have not first declared the patient at maximum medical improvement?

WHAT IS MAINTENANCE CARE?

Maintenance /Preventive Care (Mercy): Appropriate professionally acceptable treatment usually for a chronic condition or after completion of therapeutic or supportive care, directed at a symptomatically stationary condition with anticipation of maintaining optimal body function, and usually provided on some routine or regular basis. Continued treatment after a patient has reached MMI, resolution, and/or stabilization of a condition would constitute maintenance type care in nature.

WHAT IS SUPPORTIVE CARE?

Supportive care (Mercy): Treatment/care for patients having reached MMI, in whom periodic trials of withdrawal from care fail to sustain previous therapeutic gains that would otherwise progressively deteriorate. Supportive care follows appropriate application of active and passive care including lifestyle modifications. It is appropriate when rehabilitative and/or functional restorative and alternative care options, including home-based self-care and lifestyle modifications, have been considered and attempted. Supportive care may be inappropriate when it interferes with other appropriate primary care, or when the risk of supportive care outweighs its benefits, i.e., physician dependence, somatization, illness behavior, and secondary gain.

Supportive care (NCRS): Supportive treatment is to be considered the continuation of therapeutic treatment once the patient has reached a point of maximum improvement, while experiencing some permanent impairment. Supportive treatment is considered appropriate when there is documented failure of clinical trial of withdrawal, appropriate alternate forms of treatment including home-based self-treatment have been considered and/or attempted, and the supportive treatment does not interfere with any other primary treatment that the patient may be receiving.

WHAT ARE THE KEY DIFFERENCES BETWEEN SUPPORTIVE CARE AND MAINTENANCE CARE?

There are a few key differences between maintenance care and supportive care that distinguish the two. Maintenance care is typically rendered on a regular basis to help maintain optimal body function and usually when there is little or no active symptomatology or the symptoms have become stationary. Supportive care is not typically rendered on a pre-scheduled or routine basis. Supportive care is usually rendered on an "as needed" basis solely in response to symptomatic exacerbations. This may vary from case to case. The patient may only require treatment for a few exacerbation's per year but the treatment required to treat these exacerbations is at the frequency at three times a week for two weeks.

WHAT ARE THE CRITERIA FOR SUPPORTIVE CARE?

CRITERIA FOR SUPPORTIVE CARE

1. The patient must be at Maximum Medical Improvement.
2. Objective evidence of a permanent injury. Ancillary diagnostic tests must correlate with clinical examination findings due to the false positive rates with some diagnostic tests.
3. There must be documented trials of treatment withdrawal which resulted in deterioration of a patient's condition. A trial of withdrawal is having the patient go a specified period of time without treatment and then reexamining the patient to see if there has been a deterioration of their clinical status. The doctor would examine the patient and the patient would go one month or more months before they are reexamined. No in-office treatment is rendered during this time. The examination findings are compared to see if there was an improvement or deterioration on the part of the patient. This procedure can again be repeated. Failure of the patient to maintain previous therapeutic improvement would qualify them for supportive care if the other criteria are met. You may also release a patient from care and they continue to return to receive palliative care for symptomatic exacerbations. If the patient meets the

other criteria, then they would qualify for supportive care. A conditional release (to be covered later) may also be used to show a deterioration of the clinical status without treatment and help justify the need for continued care.

4.   Alternative treatments must have been tried.

5.   Care is typically rendered on a PRN ("as needed") basis in response to an exacerbation. The visits should not be prescheduled.

6.   Frequency typically should not exceed one or two times per month but this may vary depending on the specifics of the case.

7.   Supportive care does not interfere with any other primary care.

Since the typical frequency is one to two times per month, I would not recommend having the patient schedule every other week. If a reviewer picks up on this (and I'm sure they will), they may deny treatment because it is "prescheduled" and would be considered more of a maintenance type of care. Remember, supportive care is rendered in response to symptomatic exacerbations and is not pre-scheduled.

Long-term supportive care is treatment to return the patient to pre-exacerbation status and improve or maintain activities of daily living and/or work status. Mental attitude may be improved and the patient's reliance on medication is decreased. Supportive care may also be rendered as a preventative to surgery. The doctor must understand the psychosocial involvement in chronic pain and avoid physician dependence as much as possible by advocating active involvement on the part of the patient.

WHAT IS A CONDITIONAL RELEASE ?

A conditional release is when the doctor releases a patient on the condition that the patient does not experience an exacerbation of symptoms in a specified period of time. Recurrences of musculoskeletal complaints are commonly seen in practice. If you permanently release a patient and they suffer a recurrence one week after you released them, it may be difficult to convince the insurance company that it is still the same injury. The doctor would release the patient and specify a time frame, usually not more than 60 days. If the patient does not have a recurrence, they will be considered permanently released. A new injury would certainly not qualify. The recurrence would be only due to the patient's activities of daily living and not a new mechanism of injury. The typical treatment would be relatively minor to resolve the patient's recurrence.

For example, Mr. Smith's subjective and objective findings have improved. Today he will be given a conditional release. If he has a recurrence of symptoms in the next thirty days he is to call our office and return for care. If he does not require care within the thirty day period, we will consider him permanently released from treatment of his injuries sustained on 1/11/91.

Using a conditional release will be a benefit to both the doctor and patient. I am sure that most of us have treated a patient and released them from care only to have the patient return for a symptomatic exacerbation. If this happens in the

Workers' Compensation or auto insurance system, there is a likelihood that treatment beyond when the patient was released will be denied by a peer reviewer. This scenario can be avoided by using a conditional release.

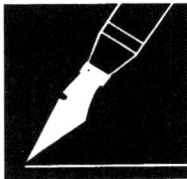

CHAPTER THREE

NEUROMUSCULAR TERMINOLOGY

It may seem very basic to cover some of these terms but it is necessary to review these in order to properly form a diagnosis and treatment frequency spectrum. You must always know what phase of treatment the patient is in so that you may pick the most appropriate form of treatment. If you diagnose a moderate sprain/strain injury and are performing a resistive rehabilitation protocol three days after the injury, is this appropriate? If you are doing this to a patient, they are either not a severe injury or you are creating further tearing and injury. This scenario is sometimes seen when reviewing a case.

GRADES OF STRAIN

1. *Grade 1 or Mild*
    - This is typically produced by a forceful stretch or trauma. A mild injury results in minimal inflammation and disruption of muscle fibers.
    - There is little swelling and edema present.
    - These injuries may not even present to the doctor for treatment.

2. *Grade 2 or Moderate*
    - A forceful overstretch or contraction results in muscle fibers being torn and hemorrhage being present. Swelling, edema, spasm, and functional loss will be present but there will not be complete disruption of muscle fibers.

3. *Grade 3 or Severe*
    - This will have all of the signs of an inflammatory response (edema, pain, redness, and swelling.) This injury usually results from a violent trauma. A complete loss of function is usually seen due to the tearing of the muscle or tendon. A muscle spasm is present to protect the injured area from further injury.

GRADES OF SPRAIN

1. *Grade 1 or Mild*
    - These injuries result in minimal tearing of ligamentous fibers. No functional loss is present and the inflammation and edema are minimal.

2. *Grade 2 or Moderate*
    - A greater degree of tear will occur to the ligaments and partial functional loss will occur. Pain, edema, and inflammation is seen with this injury.
3. *Grade 3 or Severe*
    - A complete loss of function results from a complete ligamentous tear or disruption. This injury is characterized by edema, inflammation, and hemorrhage and may requires surgical intervention. This may also lead to the development of degenerative changes and permanent instability.

PHASES OF TREATMENT

1. *Stage 1/ Acute (48-72 hours)*
    - History, examination, x-rays, and other ancillary diagnostic tests
    - Immobilization usually not to exceed 3-4 days.,
    - Cryotherapy
    - Microcurrent
    - High volt galvanic
    - Interferential
    - Activity and work modifications.
    - Orthopedic supports
    - Spinal adjustments
2. *Stage 2/Repair (48 Hours to 6 weeks)*
    - Superficial or deep heat.
    - Adjustments/manipulation
    - Nerve or muscle stimulation
    - Soft tissue procedures
    - Intersegmental traction
    - Passive exercises
    - Reexaminations: Evaluation of a patient at intervals of weeks or months for the purpose of assessing the need for continued care, modified care, cessation of care,or referral. The examinations are used to determine patient progress and to modify treatment accordingly.
    - Frequency and therapy utilization decreases according to the patient's progress.
3. *Stage 3/Remodeling (6 weeks to 12 months)*
    - Treatment is switched from passive care to a more active form of treatment
    - In-office or home exercise protocols
    - Spinal adjustments/manipulations
    - Muscle stimulation

INTENSITY GRADING (AMA GUIDES)

1. *Minimal:* The symptoms or signs are annoying but have not been documented medically to cause appreciable diminution in an individual's capacity to carry out daily activities.

2. *Slight:* The symptoms or signs are tolerated by the individual and have been documented medically to cause some diminution in an individual's capacity to carry out activities of daily living.

3. *Moderate:* The symptom or signs have been documented medically to cause serious diminution in an individual's capacity to carry out activities of daily living.

4. Marked: The symptoms or signs preclude carrying out activities of daily living.

The patient's history and examination should correlate with these definitions. It would be inappropriate to say the intensity is moderate or marked if they are able to work their full employment and are able to carry out their activities of daily living. By definition, these terms indicate that there is an inability to perform the activities of daily living.

FREQUENCY GRADING (AMA GUIDES)

1. *Intermittent:* The symptoms or signs have been documented medically to occur less than one-fourth (25%) of the time when the patient is awake.

2. *Occasional:* The symptoms or signs have been documented medically to occur between one-fourth and one-half (25%-50%) of the time when the patient is awake.

3. *Frequent:* The symptoms and signs have been documented to occur between one-half and three-fourths (50%-75%) of the time when the patient is awake.

4. *Constant:* The symptoms and signs occur between three-fourths and all (75%-100%) of the time when the patient is awake.

PATIENT ENCOUNTER DEFINITIONS

During the scope of a review you may be asked to comment on the procedure code or the complexity of the examination needed for a particular condition. You would first make sure that there was sufficient documentation to support the billing code. It would not be appropriate to bill for a comprehensive examination if there were only ten words in the records and one or two orthopedic tests done on that particular date of service. This is actually not too uncommon when doing a file review. The patient encounter definitions include:

1. *Problem Focused*
   - Single area involved
   - Transient in nature
   - Immediate identity of problem
   - No restriction of activities

2. *Expanded*
   - One or two areas involved
   - No diagnostic challenge
   - None to minor restrictions
   - Condition improving
   - Full recovery anticipated

3. *Detailed*
   - Multiple areas involved
   - Acute condition improving
   - Light activity restrictions
   - Slight exacerbation
   - Prognosis uncertain

4. *Comprehensive*
   - Multiple areas involved
   - Acute exacerbations to same or new area
   - New incident involved
   - Restricted activities in work and/or activities of daily living
   - Added complications
   - Referral or second opinion suggested

MEDICAL DECISION MAKING

1. *Minimal*
   - Does not require the presence of a physician
   - A single area is involved
   - PT/procedure performed by non-physician
   - Chronic or rehabilitation state of care
   - No risk

2. *Self-Limited/Minor*
   - One to two areas involved
   - Signs and symptoms decreasing in severity and symptoms
   - No new complaints
   - Decreasing treatment plan

3. *Low to Moderate*
   - Single area acute, or multiple areas with moderate signs and symptoms, yet decreasing in severity
   - Slight restrictions in work and/or activities of daily living
   - Decreased treatment

4. *Moderate to High*
   - Multiple areas involved
   - Signs and symptoms acute
   - Restrictions and preclusions in work and/or activities of daily living
   - Acute aggravation or new conditions involved
   - Added complications
   - Intense or increased treatment plan
   - Home treatment added
   - Second opinion or referral

STAGING OF THE EPISODE (TIME FRAMES)

These terms are for time frames and not to be confused with the healing stages of soft tissue injury and repair to be covered in Chapter 12. These definitions vary somewhat depending on which text or reference is used.

1. *Acute*
   - The word acute in treatment time protocols applies to the first 6 weeks to 8 weeks of clinical management. These conditions may present with all of the classic signs of inflammation and this term indicates a condition of recent onset or recurrence. This is most often of short duration and most cases are self-limiting and usually resolved in 6-8 weeks. The Quebec study (1987) defines this stage as 0-7 days.

2. *Acute exacerbation of a chronic condition*
   - This term describes a chronic condition that has been present for some time but has recently flared up for no apparent reason or has recently been reinjured.

3. *Subacute*
   - This describes conditions that have persisted beyond the initial 6-8 week period but have not been present for a sufficient enough time to be considered chronic. This time frame typically lasts from 6 to 16 weeks. The signs of acute injury have diminished but the symptoms have not diminished. The Quebec Study defines this stage as lasting 7 days to 7 weeks.

4. *Chronic*
   - This describes a musculoskeletal disorder lasting longer than 12 to 16 weeks without remission. By definition, chronic conditions are not self-limiting and may be very challenging to treat. These may result from acute injuries that have received little or improper treatment.
   - It is widely accepted that 90% of musculoskeletal injuries resolve within 3-4 months and that those injuries that go on to become chronic have a poor long term prognosis. The 10% of conditions that become chronic account for approximately 80% of all expenditures. The Quebec Study defines this stage as conditions lasting longer than 7 weeks.

GLOSSARY OF TERMS

INTERCONNECTING TERMINOLOGY

Each doctor should become familiar with these terms. They are important when constructing a clinical impression and also in medico-legal proceedings. Some of the terms have very similar meanings and you should become familiar with the differences. The terms include

- *Accompanying:* Denotes companionship with, but not dependency upon or necessarily closely joined; that is, may be co-existing but possibly independent

- *Associated:* Closely joined, but not necessarily dependent upon

- *Attendant:* Following as consequential

- *Concomitant:* That which accompanies or is attendant with

- *Concurrent:* Occurring at the same time or in conjunction with; however has no direct relationship

- *Consequent:* Following as a result of

- *Episodic:* Occurring, appearing or changing at irregular intervals, usually does not have a pattern to its reoccurrence.

- *Intermittent:* Returning or recurrent condition that has a pattern to its occurrence; where a period of time has not occurred showing a resolution of the clinical status

- *Predisposed:* To give a tendency toward.

- *Preexisting:* To exist before, but not necessarily giving a tendency to

    When traumatized may be
    - *Aggravated:* To further excite, increase or irritate a preexisting condition
    - *Activated:* To excite a dormant condition into becoming symptomatic expressive
    - *Accelerated:* A trauma which hastens the pathology or effects of pre-existing condition

- *Recurrent:* Returning or reoccurrence after a period of time showing a resolution of the clinical status between episodes

- *Resultant:* Resulting from something else

TISSUE DESCRIPTION

MUSCLE/TENDON

1. *Strain:* Damage to muscular or tendon tissue as a result of a sudden forceful contraction or a violent overstretching usually occurring in midrange of motion on effort

   History
   - Incident and then progressively gets worse
   - Isotonic contraction that was too great or prolonged isometric contraction
   - Due to a blow or overstretching

   Clinical Features
   - Contraction causes pain. O'Donaghue's test differentiates strain from sprain
   - Pain on resistive motion over the affected muscle
   - Pain on stretching of the affected muscle
   - Pain on moderate digital pressure to the affected muscle
   - Alteration of palpatory textures (swelling, muscle spasm, or hypertonicity)
   - Initial injury often described as a sting and gets worse with time
   - If damage is only done to the fascia, the proper term is **myofascial strain**

2. *Tendonitis:* A general term used to describe a noninfectious inflammatory process of tendon or tendon muscle attachment

   History
   - Can be due to repetitive microtrauma or a single large strain injury

   Clinical Features
   - Similar features as strain
   - Local swelling and palpatory tenderness

3. *Myositis:* This term indicates inflammation to the belly of a muscle following an acute injury such as a strain injury

4. *Myofascitis:* Inflammation of a muscle or fascia. This refers particularly to the fascia insertion of the muscle to the bone

   History
   - A sequel to a strain injury that is found. Usually found in the subacute and/or chronic stage

   Clinical Features
   - Small nodules within the fascial sheaths that are very sensitive.
   - These conditions are sensitive to colds and drafts

5. *Myofibrositis or myofascial fibrositis:* Inflammation of the perimysium of the muscle

   History
   - An injury several years prior that was not adequately treated or a repetitive strain injury

   Clinical Features
   - This is a chronic injury where there has been tissue replaced with fibrous scar tissue
   - Characterized by stiffness and rigidity in the injured area
   - These may be very persistent and painful
   - Muscle contraction or overstretching may result in "cramping" of the muscle
   - Palpatory pressure being applied to the muscle results in increased pain

6. *Myalgia*
   - Pain in a muscle or muscles
   - Muscle spasm
   - A sudden involuntary contraction of muscle or group of muscles caused by any injury to the affected area. Spasm is accompanied by pain and interference with function.

7. *Splinting Muscle Spasm*
   - A rigidity of muscles occurring as a means to protect a body part and avoid pain by movement.

JOINTS/LIGAMENTS

1. *Sprain:* An injury to ligamentous tissue due to an over-stretching of the tissue occurring at the extremes of joint motion only.

   History
   - Initial injury that progressively gets worse
   - An over-stretching that results in a concomitant strain
   - A sudden unexpected motion or loss of protective muscle tone due to fatigue results in overstretching of ligamentous tissue and possibly the joint capsule

   Clinical Features
   - Pain on both active and passive motion
   - Muscle contraction may cause little or no pain
   - Pain and swelling localized to the site of the ligament
   - A severe injury may result in hypermobility and instability.

2. *Articular sprain:* Entrapment of capsular tissue

History
- Immediate sharp pain on motion (Usually rotary)

Clinical Features
- Antalgic
- Motion increases local pain
- No significant swelling
- Marked decrease of ranges of motion, especially to affected side
- Only slight pain on isometric muscle contraction
- Associated splinting spasms (protective mechanisms)
- Responds very well to proper manipulation

3. *Arthralgia*
- This is pain in any joint

4. *Bursitis*
- Inflammation of a bursa. This can involve both superficial or deep bursae

5. *Synovitis*
- Inflammation of synovial membrane that is often associated with swelling.

6. *Capsulitis*
- Inflammation of joint capsule and internal joint ligaments
- Usually follows a sprain injury and is commonly referred to as a facet syndrome
- Extension will cause increased pain
- Scar tissue formation can result in adhesive capsulitis

7. *Periarticular fibrosis*
- Fibrotic changes surrounding a joint that is usually the chronic sequel to an improperly treated sprain or joint injury.

NERVES

1. *Radiculitis*
- Inflammation of a nerve root of a spinal nerve
- Symptoms travel in a dermatomal pattern which can result in
  - Pain—Hyperesthesia
  - Hypoesthesia—Paresthesia
  - From DJD, disc protrusion, adhesions, capsulitis, etc.

2. *Radiculalgia:* Pain due to a diseased spinal nerve root. This extends only a short distance from the involved nerve root

3. *Radiculoneuralgia:* Pain in a dermatomal pattern extending down the course of a nerve from the involved nerve root.

4. *Radiculoneuritis:* Diminished reflex, muscle weakness, or muscle atrophy associated with the above.

5. *Neuralgia*
   - Pain from a peripheral nerve covering the area of distribution of that particular nerve. This covers a greater area than the radiculo conditions.
   - These do not follow a dermatomal pattern and result in no muscle atrophy.

6. *Neuropathy:* The same as the above but in the subacute stage. This is characterized by possible reflex changes, muscle weakness, pain, and paresthesia.

7. *Neuritis*
   - Peripheral nerve inflammation and degeneration
   - Sharp and continuous pain is present
   - Decreased or absent sensation, muscle weakness or atrophy may be seen

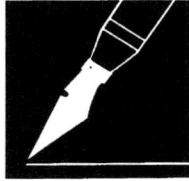

CHAPTER • FOUR

DOCUMENTATION

OVERVIEW

Adequate documentation is necessary in today's health care system. Proper record keeping is needed to receive payment from third party payers more than ever before. It seems to be more common for a doctor to be judged by the quality of records he/she keeps rather than his/her clinical skills. Record keeping in Chiropractic was never a concern at one time because third party payers did not cover Chiropractic services like they do today. Record keeping in Chiropractic seems to have lagged behind other health care professions. It is important to keep quality records due to the growing trend of utilization management and review.

WHAT IS THE PURPOSE OF HEALTH CARE RECORDS?

There are several purposes for health care records. Health care records document the specific treatment that was rendered and allow for utilization review. Health care records are also very important in malpractice and personal injury cases. Adequate records do not stop a claim being brought against a doctor, but they are necessary for a defense against a malpractice claim.

Health care records also document the injuries received following specific accidents. In some states, personal injury cases do not go to court until several years after the injury. This may be years after you have last seen the patient, so it is very important to have good records to look back on so that you are able to comment about the case.

Health care records are also used to communicate treatment and results with other health care providers. This will allow for better patient care by allowing concurrent or referral providers access to previous treatment and results. If the patient moves out of the area, they can take a copy of their records and give them to their new doctor and experience no interruption in their care.

Progress notes and examinations are the basis for future report writing. Records should be reasonably complete and contain information that accurately reflects the patient's clinical status. As a health care provider, you should try to obtain pertinent information from other health care professionals. A description of treatment, treatment results, and diagnostic tests from other providers can be of value when making future clinical decisions.

ALL RECORDS SHOULD REMAIN CONFIDENTIAL UNLESS THE PATIENT AUTHORIZES THEIR RELEASE. You should be familiar with the statutes governing retention of patient records in the state or territory you are practicing in. These statutes may vary slightly from state to state.

PROPER USE AND MAINTENANCE OF RECORDS

1. Use legible handwriting

2. Anyone entering information, other than the attending doctor, must sign name (or initial).

3. Use blue or black ink. You can use red for positives.

4. Have name, date, and case number on each page.

5. Correct an error by drawing one line through it, putting date and initials. Do not use whiteout!

6. Additions: Sign and date.

7. If file gets too big, you can start an archival file. This is done by putting the older records in a file that is kept in a location other than where the files are typically put. You must also make a notation in the current file that there is an archival file. For example: Mrs. Smith has treated with you for ten years. Her file is six inches thick and takes up a lot of space in your file rack. You could keep the most recent two to three years of records, plus any ancillary diagnostic tests or other important information, in a file and use it as your "active" file. The rest of the records you put in a separate file and place it in a storage area.

INTERNAL DOCUMENTATION

These are records that are generated within the chiropractor's office. This includes all forms, examinations, x-rays, laboratory tests, correspondence, etc. Phone messages and conversations must also be included in the patient's file. This area also includes the treatment plan devised for the management of the patient.

The treatment plan documents the particular approach to the management of the case (adjustment, modalities, exercise, lifestyle changes, etc.). This also includes plans for outside referrals, diagnostic tests, patient education and reassessment.

Example of a treatment plan: Treatment will consist of spinal adjustments for joint fixation, cryotherapy to lumbar spine 15 min. for pain and spasm, and myofascial release to the lumbar spine to decrease adhesions. Treatment will be at the frequency of three times per week for four weeks at which time the patient will be reevaluated.

Example: Treatment will consist of spinal adjustments, interferential, and myofascial release at the frequency of three times a week for two weeks. If there is no response to our treatment in this time, we will order an MRI to determine the exact location and extent of the disc herniation. Should the patient's clinical status deteriorate, he will be referred for neurosurgical evaluation.

WHAT IS A REFERRAL?

Referral (Mercy): The direction of a patient to another health care professional or institution for evaluation, consultation, or care.

The referral may be intra- or interprofessional. Intraprofessional referrals would be to another chiropractor better suited to treat a patient's chiropractic needs. A interprofessional referral would be to another health care professional for concurrent care, consultation, emergency care or for conditions outside the scope of chiropractic care. Each referral should have a rationale such as a nonresponsive patient to chiropractic care, suspicion of an underlying pathology or condition not within the scope of chiropractic or a progressive neurologic deficit.

WHAT IS MANAGEMENT?

Management (Mercy): A plan of action for the treatment of the patient in accordance with diagnosis, progress, and expectations of outcome.

EXTERNAL DOCUMENTATION

All of the records that are generated from outside the doctor's office. A reasonable attempt should be made to obtain pertinent health care records and diagnostic findings from other health care providers. These would include records from specialists, concurrent or referral health care providers, diagnostic tests, letters from insurance carriers, attorneys, etc.

CHART/FILE ORGANIZATION

All records should be kept in chronological order and should never be back dated or altered. This statement does not need an explanation!

All of the information in the records should be enough to provide subsequent care. In other words, another chiropractor should be able to understand your notes enough to provide care for your patient in a similar manner.

All records should be written neatly, organized, and complete. "A physician shall maintain medical records for patients which accurately, legibly, and completely reflect the evaluation and treatment of the patient" (Section 16.95 of Pa. Medical Records statute).

The use of nonstandard abbreviations should be accompanied by a legend and the patient's name should appear on all pages of the records. One of the most common mistakes is not supplying a key when the doctor uses nonstandard abbreviations. Remember, another doctor should be able to understand your notes enough to provide care for your patient. If you are having a case reviewed, your treatment could be denied if your records cannot be interpreted by the reviewer. Substandard or inadequate documentation is a common reason for denial of care during a utilization review.

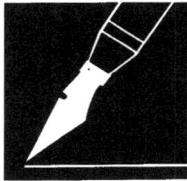

CHAPTER • FIVE

INITIAL HISTORY AND INTAKE INFORMATION

Information gathered during the initial patient interview and from intake forms is very important. This information helps lay the foundation for treatment and justification for diagnostic tests and/or concurrent care. It is recommended that only those people with the proper training be allowed to gather historical information. Obtaining information from patients is a skill in itself and should be done only by those individuals who have had adequate instruction and experience.

Following are a few items that can be asked on the history questionnaires. An example of an intake form is also provided in this chapter. Behind each item listed below is a brief explanation about the importance of acquiring this information:

- *Age?* Low back pain is increased with age.

- *Married? Single? Divorced? Separated?* There is an increased incidence of back pain with poor life and job satisfaction and loneliness.

- *Years employed at current occupation?* Employees at greatest risk for injury were those on the job for the least amount of time.

- *Education?* (Formal education and back related disability, Spine 1995) This study compared the education level of employees and found that those employees in the study who completed 12 years or less of schooling worked in jobs that were more physically demanding. These employees also had higher depression scores, were more often obese and more likely to smoke. Employees who had more than 13 years of schooling worked more in professional occupations and had less disability and a greater decline in their disability.

VERTEBROBASILAR TESTING

This is part of the physical examination often overlooked by many chiropractors. I have reviewed several hundreds of cases and have seen vertebrobasilar testing done in only a few of them. The following historical information should be gathered in an attempt to evaluate for possible vertebrobasilar insufficiency. Remember, there are several parts to a complete assessment but we will only cover the history in this text. The following are risk factors which may be associated with a higher incidence of vertebrobasilar injury following cervical spine manipulation. The questions are arranged in two groups as follows:

1. Have you ever been diagnosed or been told you have...
    *   high blood pressure?
    *   hardening of the arteries?
    *   diabetes?
    *   heart or blood vessel disease?
    *   bone spurs on the neck?
    *   whiplash injury?
    *   Have any of your relatives suffered a stroke?
    *   Did you ever smoke? When?
    *   Women only: Have you ever taken oral contraceptives?

2. Have you had any of the following symptoms for even a short or temporary duration within the last year?
    *   Blurred vision
    *   Double vision
    *   Diminished or partial loss of vision in one or both eyes
    *   Complete loss of vision in one or both eyes
    *   Ringing, buzzing, or any noise in the ears
    *   Slurred speech or other speech problems
    *   Difficulty swallowing
    *   Dizziness
    *   Temporary lack of understanding
    *   Loss of consciousness, even momentary blackouts
    *   Numbness or loss of sensation in face, arms, hands, fingers or legs
    *   Any other abnormal or loss of sensation in any other part of the body
    *   Weakness, clumsiness, or strength loss in face, arms, hands, fingers, or legs
    *   Sudden collapse without loss of consciousness

These questions may be placed on intake forms or asked by the doctor directly. If they are placed on intake forms, the examiner should review them with the patient to make sure they were answered completely and accurately. Some of these questions, particularly in the first section, give you an idea of the overall health status of the patient.

WHAT IS A CHIEF COMPLAINT?

The chief complaint is the reason for the visit. It is a concise statement describing the symptom, problem, or condition.

WHAT IS HISTORY OF THE PRESENT ILLNESS?

A chronological description of the development of the patient's present illness from the first sign and/or symptom to the present.

WHAT ARE THE 8 PARAMETERS OF THE CHIEF COMPLAINT?

This is the most basic portion of a history. These questions can be later expanded on according to the patient's response. The 8 parameters of the chief complaint include the following:

1. Date of onset
2. Mode of onset (did anything cause or contribute)
3. Location of Pain
4. Type of pain
5. Frequency of pain
6. Exacerbations and remissions (what makes better and worse)
7. Relationship to other systems
8. Prior treatment and results

History taking is a skill. If you need to work on this area, then do so. Use your staff to do mock cases and practice. The following is an example of a basic history. Are all of the components there?

> Mrs. Smith presents with a chief complaint of low back pain. She points to the lower lumbar spine and states the pain started suddenly yesterday while lifting a basket of laundry. Mrs. Smith says the pain is a sharp and severe pain that radiates down the posterior aspect of her left leg to the foot. She states "my left foot is numb." She has tried Motrin and moist heat with no improvement. Sitting for long periods increased her pain and nothing seems to help. She has had no professional care for this problem and denies any bowel or bladder involvement.

The above example is similar to what we may see in practice. This history is not extremely long but contains a lot of important information. Doctors sometimes get the proper information from the patient but have difficulty writing the information down. Complete sentences are used so that the history is easy to read and follow. Remember, there will be several people looking at your records and most of them have had no chiropractic training. These include insurance company representatives, case managers, and law firm employees.

OPQRST

This is another pneumonic used for initial history taking. Can you see how it compares to the 8 parameters?

O   Onset—Gradual or Sudden
P   Palliative-Better/Worse
Q   Quality—Sharp, Deep, Dull, Aching
R   Radiation or Localized
S   Severity—Slight, Mild, Moderate, Severe
T   Time—Rare 10%, Intermittent 25%, Occasional 50%, Frequent 75%, Constant 100%

Confidential Case History

Please Print   Dr. Mr. Mrs. Ms. Miss.   Patient#_____

Name:_____ Home#: (   )_____ Work#: (   )_____

Address:_____ City:_____ State:_____ Zip:_____

SS#:_____ Date of Birth:_____ Age:_____ Sex M F

Occupation:_____ Employer:_____ Yrs. Employed:_____

Marital Status:_____ Spouse's Name:_____ Spouse's Occupation:_____

If retired, former occupation:_____ Education level obtained:_____

Primary Care Physician (name, address and telephone):_____
_____

NOTE: If you're on Medicare, please show your card to the receptionist.
_____

MAIN COMPLAINT: Why are you here today? Be specific with location:_____
_____

1. When did it start?   Date: _____

2. How did it start? Explain _____

3. Work-related injury? Y   N   Auto accident? Y   N   Injury at home? Y   N
   Injury elsewhere? Y   N

4. Does it radiate to any other part of your body? Y   N   Where?_____

5. Did it begin gradually or suddenly? _____

6. How would you describe the intensity? (mild, moderate, severe) _____

7. Describe your pain (dull, sharp, burning, numbness, soreness, stiffness) other _____

8. Has your problem been getting better, worse or about the same? _____

9. Does your condition come and go or is it all the time?_____

10. What makes your symptoms better?_____

11. What makes your symptoms worse?_____

12. Have you tried home remedies? Y   N   What?_____

13. What doctors have you seen and what tests have been done for your condition?_____

14. Have you had anything like this before? Y   N   Details_____

15. Have there been any other changes in any body functions? Y   N   Details_____

16. Has your condition affected your daily activities in any way? Y   N   Explain_____

17. Have you been unable to work as a result of your current problem?_____

18. Do you have any other problems that you would like the doctors to evaluate?_____

**MARK THE AREAS ON YOUR BODY
WHERE YOU HAVE SYMPTOMS.**

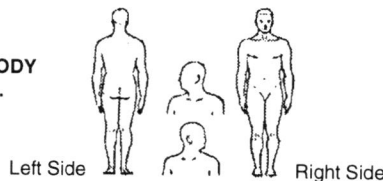

Left Side   Right Side

Past History:

1. Have you had any of the following childhood diseases: (circle) Measles, rubella, chickenpox, mumps, scarlet fever, rheumatic fever, tuberculosis. Other?_____

2. Have you been diagnosed with any other conditions?   Y   N   Explain:_____

3. Are you under a doctor's care presently for any type of health problem?_____

4. Have you had any broken bones?   Y   N   Which ones?_____

5. Have you ever had any past significant auto accidents, work injuries or falls?   Y   N   When?_____

6. Are you taking any medication? Please list. _____

7. Have you ever undergone any type of surgery?   What and when?_____

8. Do you smoke, drink alcohol or use recreational drugs?_____

9. Do you have any allergies?_____

10. Do any diseases run in your family?_____

HAVE YOU BEEN DIAGNOSED OR
BEEN TOLD YOU HAVE THE FOLLOWING?

Y	N	High blood pressure
Y	N	Hardening of the arteries
Y	N	Diabetes
Y	N	Heart or blood vessel disease
Y	N	Bone spurs on the neck
Y	N	Whiplash injury
Y	N	Any relatives ever suffer a stroke?
Y	N	Blurred vision
Y	N	Double vision
Y	N	Do you currently smoke?
Y	N	Have you smoked in the past?

MEN ONLY:
Date of last prostate exam: _____

Difficulty with urination?_____

Excessive urination?_____

WOMEN ONLY:
Do you experience any of the following symptoms?

Y	N	Do you take birth control pills? How long?_____
Y	N	Menstrual pain
Y	N	Cramping
Y	N	Irregularity Date of last period _____
Y	N	Are you pregnant? How long?_____

HAVE YOU HAD ANY OF THESE FOLLOWING SYMPTOMS
FOR EVEN A SHORT OR TEMPORARY DURATION WITHIN
THE LAST YEAR?

Y	N	Slurred speech or other speech problems
Y	N	Difficulty swallowing
Y	N	Dizziness
Y	N	Temporary lack of understanding
Y	N	Loss of consciousness, even momentary blackouts
Y	N	Numbness or loss of sensation in the face, arms, hands, fingers, or legs
Y	N	Any other abnormal or loss of sensation in any other part of your body
Y	N	Weakness, clumsiness, or strength loss in the face, arms, hands, fingers, or legs
Y	N	Sudden collapse without loss of consciousness
Y	N	Diminished or partial loss of vision in one or both eyes
Y	N	Hearing loss in one or both ears

ATTENTION- Payment is to be made at the time of the visit unless prior arrangements have been made with this office. Also a 24-Hour notice is necessary to cancel an appointment, and you may be responsible for payment of a missed appointment.

I hereby consent to any procedures or treatments necessary for treatment of any condition as deemed reasonable by the attending doctor.

Patient signature _____ Date_____

OTHER QUESTIONS

Have you ever been diagnosed with a particular condition?

Have you ever had any broken bones?

Have you had any injuries?

Have you had any surgeries?

What medications are you currently taking?

Do you wear heel lifts or other supports?

REVIEW OF SYSTEMS

General Constitutional symptoms: Fever, chills, fatigue, etc.

Skin

Musculoskeletal

Head: Eyes, ears, nose and throat

Endocrine

Respiratory

Cardiovascular

Gastrointestinal

Genitourinary

Psychiatric

PAST MEDICAL HISTORY

General health

Childhood and adult illnesses

Surgeries

Medications

Allergies

These questions help give you an idea of the patients overall health status. Metabolic conditions, smoking, drug use, multiple injuries, obesity, medications, and psychological disorders all will complicate treatment.

BACK MUSCLE INJURY AFTER POSTERIOR LUMBAR SPINE SURGERY
Spine 1994

Atrophy of the sacrospinalis muscles and erector spinae muscles is common following posterior spine surgery. Low back pain that persists following a surgery may be attributed to trauma in the paravertebral muscles following surgery.(It is very important that you assess for a surgical history prior to rendering chiropractic care. This may not preclude you from rendering care, but will most likely lead to special management considerations.)

FAMILY HISTORY

Health of parents and siblings. If deceased, what was the cause of death? Certain illnesses such as diabetes, heart disease, etc. may have a family predisposition.

PERSONAL AND SOCIAL HISTORY

Personal information: Married, divorced/separated, hobbies, interests, etc.

Habits: diet, sleeping, drugs, exercise.

Military record

Education level attained.

OCCUPATIONAL HISTORY

Describe job. Exposure to jolting or jarring forces.

Does it involve bending or twisting at the waist repeatedly for extended periods of times?

Have you ever worked where you were exposed to toxic metals, gases, fumes, dust, extreme temperatures?

Have you ever received any permanent impairments or work restrictions?

Have you had any previous Workers' Compensation claims?

Occupational history can be very important. If the patient's job is causing or complicating an injury that they are being treated for, recovery time will most likely be prolonged. Make sure this is documented in the records. Knowing a patient's job requirements is also very important when determining readiness to return to work or work restrictions.

DELAYS TO RECOVERY (MERCY)

1. Pain more than 8 days: Recovery may take 1.5 times longer.

2. Severe pain: Recovery may take up to two times longer.

3. 4-7 previous episodes: Recovery may take up to two times longer.

4. Injury superimposed on a preexisting condition (skeletal anomaly or structural pathology): May increase recovery time 1.5-2 times.

CERVICAL ACCELERATION/DECELERATION INJURIES

A history following an automobile accident can be more complex than other injuries. We will cover some of the important areas in this discussion. For an in-depth study regarding CAD injuries, I would suggest looking at the work of Foreman and Croft. They are very well-known chiropractors and have contributed a considerable amount of literature regarding automobile injuries. I would suggest that if you are dealing with automobile injuries or reviewing records for automobile cases, buy a copy of *Whiplash Injuries: The Cervical Acceleration/Deceleration Syndrome*.

IMPORTANT HISTORICAL INFORMATION REGARDING WHIPLASH TRAUMA:

1. *The type and speed of the cars involved.* This is especially important in rear-end collisions. In rear-end collisions, the acceleration achieved by the occupant's head and trunk is proportional to the acceleration achieved by the struck vehicle. The forward acceleration of the struck vehicle depends on the mass of the vehicles, velocity of the striking vehicle, road conditions, and whether brakes were applied. Cervical spine injuries are proportional to the accretion achieved by the struck vehicle and acceleration differences between the occupant's head and trunk.

2. *Road conditions and whether brakes were applied.* These deal with frictional forces that may exist between the car and road. Dry pavement and brakes being applied would increase friction between the car and road surface whereas wet pavement with no brakes applied would decrease the friction. The amount of friction between the car and the road has an influence on the amount of acceleration the occupant's head and trunk experiences, thereby increasing or decreasing the extent of the injury. Anything decreasing the forward acceleration of the struck vehicle would decrease the injury to the occupants. Was the car stopped or moving slowly? A car moving slowly will accelerate more rapidly than one that is stopped. If a car was struck on ice, there may be little damage to the car. Because the car was allowed to move forward and accelerate rapidly, there may be significant injury to the occupants.

3. *Position of the head at the time of impact.* This would determine which anatomic structures are likely to be most injured. If the occupant's head was turned at the time of a rear-end collision, there would be greater injury on the side that the head was turned. A rear-end collision with the occupant's head looking forward would result in most of the injuries being found in the axis of flexion and extension.

4. *Readiness for impact.* Anticipation of the collision may help reduce injury, whereas unawareness would increase injury. Unawareness of the impending collision would be found more commonly in rear-end collisions.

5. *Height of the headrest and size of the occupant.* Proper use of the headrest is very important in the prevention of cervical spine injuries during a vehicle collision. If the car has no headrest, my advice would be not to drive it or be very careful. Proper placement of the headrest is above the skull's center of mass. If the headrest is below the center of mass of the skull or the occupant is above average height, the headrest may act as a fulcrum and increase the injury in the hyperextension phase. Headrests should be at least at the level of the ears to help prevent extension injuries of the neck. Cervical flexion stops at the chin, lateral flexion stops at the shoulder, but there is no natural limit to cervical spine extension. Where was the person positioned in the car? Were they in the front seat or back seat? This may make a difference if the car did not have headrests for the back seat occupants.

6. *Use of seatbelts.* The use of lap and shoulder harness seatbelts does not decrease the injuries in hyperflexion/hyperextension trauma to the cervical spine. These may, in fact, enhance injuries to the cervical spine. The shoulder

that is not restricted by the shoulder harness may be injured with the occupant potentially developing shoulder complaints and/or thoracic outlet syndrome.

7. *The type of collision.* Rear-end collisions result in injuries to the structures most involved in flexion and extension. A side or oblique collision would involve flexion and extension combined with rotation and lateral flexion. Second collisions would also be important and may magnify the injuries that were received.

8. *When did the symptoms start?* Usually, the sooner the symptoms start following the injury, the more the severe the injuries are. The following acute symptoms indicate serious injury: intense nausea, frequent vomiting, pain in the cervical paraspinal muscles, torticollis, radiculitis, pounding headache, vertigo, cervical sympathetic chain symptoms (hearing loss, dizziness, nystagmus, blurred vision, pain behind eye (dilated pupil, and photophobia are examples), poor concentration, loss of memory, and emotional reactions. Loss of consciousness may indicate cerebral concussion even if there is no direct head trauma.

9. *Other Questions.* Other questions that may be asked include the location and extent of damage to the vehicles, property, approximate speed of the vehicles and whether the police were notified. Vehicle damage is not always an indicator of occupant injury.

It is not necessarily your job to "prove" that an accident occurred, but the information about the accident will give you an idea of the injuries that were received by the occupants. Some attorneys do not want doctors to get estimated speeds of the vehicles or other information because they feel this information can be later used against their client, especially if they are wrong about certain information. I am recommending gathering this information to help the treating physician make decisions about patient care and treatment management.

FACTORS AFFECTING THE OUTCOME OF WHIPLASH INJURIES:

- Symptoms or findings of arm pain or numbness
- Rear end collisions result in more disability
- Straightening or reversal of the cervical curve
- Limited range of motion combined with neurological signs and symptoms
- Spinal stenosis
- Pre-existing degenerative changes
- Symptoms developing within 12-24 hours after injury

ACUTE LOW BACK PROBLEMS IN ADULTS: ASSESSMENT AND TREATMENT
AHCPR Guideline 14

This section covers the recommended history according to guideline 14. The goal is to assess for potentially serious conditions and to help eliminate the need for special studies since it is estimated that 90% of all patients will recover spontaneously within four weeks. The complete algorithms and tables from this guideline are covered in Chapter 10.

Red flags for potential serious conditions:

* *Possible fracture:* Major trauma such as a vehicle accident or fall from height. Minor trauma or even strenuous lifting (in older or potentially osteoporotic patient).

* *Possible tumor or infection:* Age over 50 or under 20. Cancer history, recent fever, chills, or any unexplained weight loss. Recent infection, IV drug use, or immunosuppression (from steroids, transplant, or HIV). Pain that worsens when supine. Severe nighttime pain.

* *Possible cauda equina syndrome:* Saddle anesthesia, recent onset of bladder dysfunction such as urinary retention, increased frequency, or overflow incontinence. Severe or progressive neurologic deficit in the lower extremity.

OUTCOME ASSESSMENT

This section contains some of the more common examples of outcome assessment. These are used as measurements for pain and disability. There are several in use but we will cover the ones that are most commonly used in chiropractic. Patients feel comfortable rating their own perception of pain and satisfaction with treatment. These can be used to help determine the patient's progress and response to treatment. I commonly see these used inaccurately by many doctors. The treating doctor must compare these measurements with the ones that were used previously in order to determine if the patient feels improved, regressed, or the same. They are not to be done for appearance only and placed in the file without being viewed.

The first type of outcome assessment is a pain diagram. This is a self-report of the location and extent of the pain. They are used as a way patients can communicate their pain to health care professionals. There is high reliability reported for the pain diagrams. The examiner looks at the diagrams and determines whether the reported pain follows appropriate pain behavior in an anatomically correct depiction. An example of this type would be the Ransford pain drawing.

The Visual Analog Scale (VAS) is a very simple scale designed for the self-evaluation of pain intensity. The VAS requires the patient to place a mark on a continuous line to rate their pain. There is a high level of sensitivity with this type of pain scale.

BORG PAIN SCALE, 1-10

PURPOSE:

Allows the patient to rate their pain to be used for comparison with a previous score.

PATIENT DIRECTIONS:

On a scale of 1-10, place an X in your current pain level.

Normal	Low Pain	Moderate Pain	Intense Pain	Emergency
( ) 0	( ) 1	( ) 4	( ) 7	( ) 10
	( ) 2	( ) 5	( ) 8	
	( ) 3	( ) 6	( ) 9	

SCORING:

0-3

Patients at this level may be able to return to work depending on many factors.

4-5

1. Significant degree of impairment fora nonsymptom magnifying patient

2. Low level of impairment for a patient who has a low pain threshold

6-10

1. Severe pathology

2. Symptom magnification behavior

Above 10

Symptom magnification

ADVANTAGES:

The patient can rate changes in their pain for objectivity

PAIN DRAWING

Patient Name: _____ Date: _____

Borg Pain Scale: DOB: _____

On a scale of 1 to 10 place an X in your current pain level.

NORMAL	LOW PAIN	MODERATE PAIN	INTENSE PAIN	EMERGENCY
( ) 0	( ) 1	( ) 4	( ) 7	( ) 10
	( ) 2	( ) 5	( ) 8	
	( ) 3	( ) 6	( ) 9	

RANSFORD PAIN DRAWING:

To help us better understand the nature and origin of your complaints. We will ask that you carefully complete this drawing. Use the symbols listed below to detail where you hurt and how it hurts.

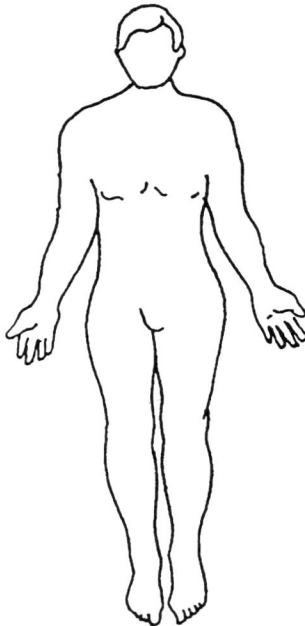

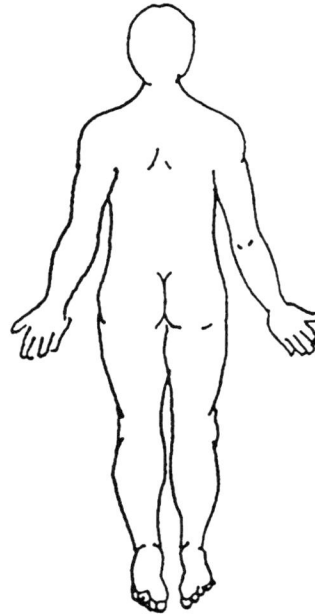

/ / / / / / / /	Dull Ache/ Throb	= = = = = = = =	Numbness
x x x x x x x x	Sharp/ Stabbing	: : : : : : : :	Tingling
BBBBBBBB	Burning	SSSSSSSS	Cramping

_____   _____
     Signature of Patient   Date

A variation of the VAS is the Numerical Rating Scale 101. The patient chooses a number between 1 and 100 to rate the severity of their pain. The Borg pain scale is a 10 point scale similar to the VAS. The Borg scale is used by having the patient rate his/her pain from 0-10 using the following definitions of the numbers: 0 = normal; 1 through 3 = low pain; 4 through 6 = moderate pain; 7 through 9 = intense pain; 10 = emergency. A patient scoring their pain from 0 to 3 should be able to return to work. A score of 4 to 5 may indicate a significant degree of impairment. A score from 6 to 10 indicates a severe pathology or symptom magnification. A score above 10 indicates symptom magnification.

The Oswestry disability questionnaire is used for low back pain. This contains various daily activities deemed relevant to low back disability. Each item is given a point value from 0-5, from top to bottom, for a potential score of 50. The score is then doubled for a total percentage score. The interpretation of the final score is provided as follows:

    0-20% Minimal ADL Disability

    20-40% Moderate ADL Disability

    40-60% Severe ADL Disability

    60-80% Crippled ADL Disability

    80-100% Symptom Magnification or Bed Bound

Waddell's examination is used to perform a rating with regard to symptom magnification. There are five categories of examination: tenderness, simulation, distraction, regional, and overreaction. There must be at least three positive categories before an assessment of symptom magnification can be made.

All of the tests previously mentioned in the section involve the patient's rating or evaluating themselves. There are other types of outcome assessment. Physiologic outcomes can also be used by the doctor to monitor patient progress. Physiologic outcomes include range of motion, muscle function, and posture to name a few. The Straight Leg Raising test and the degree at which it causes pain may also be used to monitor a patient's progress with low back disc herniations.

Standardized outcome assessments can be of value in determining maximum improvement and evaluating the effect of treatment over time. These measures also document improvement to third party payers and help quantify clinical findings. Treatment dosage, type, and duration may also be justified and modifications to treatment made with the aid of outcome measures.

OWESTRY DISABILITY QUESTIONNAIRE

Directions: This questionnaire has been designed to give the doctor information as to how your pain has affected your ability to manage in everyday life. Please circle in each section only <u>one</u> statement which most closely applies to you.

Section 1—Pain Intensity
1. I can tolerate the pain I have without having to use pain killers.
2. The pain is bad, but I can manage without taking pain killers.
3. Pain killers give complete relief from pain.
4. Pain killers give moderate relief from pain.
5. Pain killers give very little relief from pain.
6. Pain killers have no effect on the pain and I do not use them.

Section 2—Personal Care (washing, dressing, etc.)
1. I can look after myself normally without causing extra pain.
2. I can look after myself normally, but it causes extra pain.
3. It is painful to look after myself and I am slow and careful.
4. I need some help every day in most of my personal care.
5. I need help every day in most aspects of self-care.
6. I do not get dressed, wash with difficulty, and stay in bed.

Section 3—Lifting
1. I can lift heavy weights without extra pain.
2. I can lift heavy weights but it gives extra pain.
3. Pain prevents me from lifting heavy weights off the floor, but I can manage if they are conveniently positioned.
4. Pain prevents me from lifting heavy weights, but I can lift light to medium weights if they are conveniently positioned.
5. I can lift only very light weights.
6. I cannot lift or carry anything at all.

Section 4—Walking
1. Pain does not prevent me walking any distance.
2. Pain prevents me walking more than 1 mile.
3. Pain prevents me walking more than 1/2 mile.
4. Pain prevents me walking more than 1/4 mile.
5. I can only walk using a cane or crutches.
6. I am in bed most of the time and have to crawl to the toilet.

Section 5—Sitting
1. I can sit in any chair as long as I like.
2. I can only sit in my favorite chair as long as I like.
3. Pain prevents me sitting more than 1 hour.
4. Pain prevents me from sitting more than 1/2 hour.
5. Pain prevents me from sitting more than 10 minutes.
6. Pain prevents me from sitting at all.

Section 6—Standing
1. I can stand as long as I want without extra pain.
2. I can stand as long as I want but it gives me extra pain.
3. Pain prevents me from standing for more than 1 hour.
4. Pain prevents me from standing for more than 30 minutes.
5. Pain prevents me from standing for more than 10 minutes.
6. Pain prevents me from standing at all.

Section 7—Sleeping
1. Pain does not prevent me from sleeping well.
2. I can sleep well only by using tablets.
3. I have less than six hours of sleep before pain awakens me.
4. I have less than four hours sleep before pain awakens me.
5. I have less than two hours sleep before pain awakens me.
6. Pain prevents me from sleeping at all.

Section 8—Sex Life
1. My sex life is normal and causes me no extra pain.
2. My sex life is normal but causes some extra pain.
3. My sex life is nearly normal but is very painful.
4. My sex life is restricted by pain.
5. My sex life is nearly absent because of pain.
6. Pain prevents any sex life at all.

Section 9—Social Life
1. My social life is normal and gives me no extra pain.
2. My social life is normal but increases the degree of pain.
3. Pain has no significant effect on my social life apart from limiting my more energetic interests.
4. Pain restricts my social life and I do not go out as often.
5. Pain has restricted my social life to my home.
6. I have no social life because of pain.

Section 10—Traveling
1. I can travel anywhere without extra pain.
2. I can travel anywhere but it gives me extra pain.
3. Pain is bad but I manage journeys over 2 hours.
4. Pain restricts me to journeys less than 1 hour.
5. Pain restricts me to short necessary journeys under 30 minutes.
6. Pain prevents me from traveling except to the doctor or hospital.

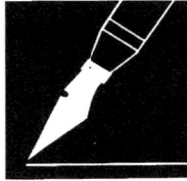

CHAPTER • SIX

PROGRESS NOTES

Progress notes are by definition a brief notation in the patient's file for each visit once management has commenced. Initial examinations and reevaluations are more comprehensive than daily progress notes. Progress notes must be sufficiently complete to provide reasonable information to a subsequent provider, insurance company, or attorney. Each visit must be dated and changes in the clinical picture, assessment, or treatment plan are noted. There will typically be less change in the clinical status from visit to visit versus monthly exam to monthly exam.

PURPOSE OF SOAP NOTES:

1. Gives progressive and sequential order to the patient's record.
2. To give a concise and coherent recording of the patient's assessment, clinical findings, and care with each patient encounter.
3. To assist the doctor in tracking the patient's response to care.
4. To identify the patient's problems and regimen of care for subsequent chiropractors, other allied health care providers, insurance providers and peer review.
5. Proof of treatment.
6. Foundation for future report writing.
7. To allow for communication with insurance carrier, other physicians, and reviewers.
8. Potential application for research.

S = SUBJECTIVE

The subjective component includes comments reported by the patient on forms, questionnaires, pain drawings, and history. These are direct quotes from the patient in response to questions asked by the doctor. This portion should reflect the patient's point of view and the patient's interpretation of their current circumstances. Examples include location and type of pain, response to treatment, and changes in activities of daily living. This information will assist in setting goals for patient treatment and determining when to modify or discontinue treatment.

O = OBJECTIVE

These are observable findings relevant to the problem. This information is used to plan patient care and justify the need for care. Examples include range of motion, reflexes, motor, visual analysis, algometer, palpation, instrumentation, muscle testing, chiropractic analysis, mensuration, ortho/neuro, diagnostic findings, lab and special testing, and psychological testing. Every few visits you should retest the positive findings. Every few weeks the doctor should retest more completely.

A = ASSESSMENT

This includes the diagnosis, response to treatment and prognosis. This area is for your professional consideration and judgment of S + O (Subjective + Objective). Short- and long-term goals are found here. Short-term goals may include: reduce pain and spasm, maintain activities of daily living, return to work, etc. Long-term goals may include increased flexibility, strength, and/or endurance; increased range of motion, return to a full-duty capacity, etc.

This section includes the doctor's impressions and interpretation. The doctor should describe his/her feelings about the status of the patient. The doctor should list a diagnosis and can modify this at any time as the clinical status of the patient changes.

Example: The patient's diagnosis is acute non-traumatic severe lumbar spine sprain/strain.

P = PLAN   P = PROCEDURES   P = PROGNOSIS

This section is where you will put the treatment plan, procedures, and sometimes the prognosis. The plan is directly related to the assessment portion of the SOAP notes. This includes diagnostic, therapeutic, and patient education plans. Future plan for referrals, therapy, reassessment, modifications of treatment, home care, and exercises are found here. The plan can be discontinued, altered, or revised as need dictates. Treatment is recorded here including frequency and duration, therapy dose and duration. Examples of treatment plans were shown previously in Chapter 4. Total and partial disability and supplies given to the patient are found here.

KEY POINTS TO SOAP NOTES:

1. Use complete sentence structure as much as possible.

2. One of your peers should be able to understand your notes well enough to treat your patient.

3. Avoid repetitive or lengthy computer generated notes. All of the notations should not be the same. Some computer generated notes have a limited vocabulary and most of the entries look the same or very similar.

4. Progress notes should be easy to follow.

STIM

S = Surgery

T = Trauma

I = Illness

M = Medication

STIM is a brief review of the patient's health status that can be done every visit, every few visits, weeks, or months. This gives information regarding any changes in the clinical history from the time you last saw the patient.

EXAMPLES OF SOAP NOTES

EXAMPLE 1 (EXAMINATION)

S: The patient presents and states " I have pain that started Monday." The patient indicates that while driving at work on Monday that he began to experience low back pain. He states that it has progressively became worse over the last two days until he came here. He states the pain is severe and "shoots down the legs." He denies trauma or injury. He points to the lower lumbar spine as the location of the pain. Sitting for long periods of time increases the pain. Coughing and sneezing increases the pain. He denies bowel or bladder involvement. He has tried ice at home with no results.

O: The patient is forward antalgic. There is a severe decrease in lumbar spine range of motion. Lower extremity reflexes are +2/4 bilaterally. Lower extremity motor is +5/5 bilaterally. Valsalva's maneuver produces localized pain at L4/5. Bechterew's test is positive on left and negative on the right. Kemp's test is positive on the right and left with localized pain at L4/5. Straight Leg Raising test is positive on left at 60 degrees with local pain at L4/5 and negative on the right. Braggard's test is negative right and left. There is joint fixation at L4/5. Spasm of lumbar paraspinal musculature. X-rays show degenerative disc disease at L4/5.

A: Acute lumbar spine segmental dysfunction complicated by degenerative disc disease. Patient has responded to similar problems in the past. Short-term goals are to decrease pain and spasm and return patient to work.

P: Treatment consisted of flexion/distraction to the lumbar spine, side posture adjustment, moist heat to lumbar spine for 15 min. to decrease spasm. The patient is to return in 2 days. If there is no significant response to care in one week we will consider MRI of the lumbar spine to rule/out central disc HNP at L4/5 that is complicated by degenerative changes.

EXAMPLE 2

S: Patient presents today with a continued complaint of low back pain that is unchanged since last visit. She continues to use cryotherapy at home as directed.

O: Tenderness and hypertonicity of the L3-5 lumbar paraspinal musculature.

A: Patient's condition unchanged

P: Treatment today consisted of spinal adjustment, interferential and massage therapy. Patient will return for follow-up care in 2 days.

EXAMPLE 3

S: LBP

O: 5L PRS

A: Same

P: Return 2 days

This example contains minimal information. Write out the words for the history and use complete sentences as much as possible. This may suffice for one visit, but if there are many visits like this, progress will be difficult to follow.

EXAMPLE 4

S: Neck pain

O: See above

A: See above

P: Continue care

Avoid using "see above" and "same as last visit." This becomes confusing and difficult to follow, especially if these notations are used on several consecutive days.

EXAMPLE 5

S: The patient presents today with a chief complaint of mild intermittent low back pain for three days. The patient states " it is starting to get tight." Patient denies trauma or injury. He denies radiating pain.

O: Lumbar range of motion is within normal limits with no pain. Straight Leg Raising test is negative right and left. Lower extremity reflexes +2/4 bilaterally. Joint fixation and tenderness at L4/5.

A: Lumbar segmental dysfunction.

P: Treatment = adjustment. Home moist heat 15 min. 1x/ day. R/S PRN

EXAMPLE 6

S: The patient stated that on today's visit that there was a slight worsening of his low back pain. He states he is feeling some improvement in his thoracic pain. There is also definite improvement in his headache but his neck pain is increased.

O: A posterior rotation subluxation with right superior deviation was noted at C2. There is an increase in the hypertonic muscular contraction in the gluteus maximus elicited on palpation.

A: Subluxations at C2, C5, T4, L4, and the left ilium

P: A two-week appointment is scheduled. An adjustment was performed to restore joint motion.

EXAMPLE 7

S: "My back and ribs are feeling better."

O: Spasm resolved in the thoracic spine. Soto Hall's test is negative.

A: Patient improving.

P: Treatment consisted of spinal adjustment, hot pack and electrical stimulation to the lumbar spine. Return appointment in one week.

All of these previous examples, except 3 and 4, would be sufficient having fulfilled the criteria for daily progress notes. Some of these examples are brief notations but contain the required elements. From my experience, if you would keep notes like these few good examples, you would be in the top half of the profession as far as progress notes are concerned.

The length of your progress notes and examinations are in relation to the complexity of the patient's history, examination findings, assessment and complicating factors. You would do a more complete examination on someone whom you have not seen in six months versus someone you saw two days ago and has not had any significant change in his or her condition.

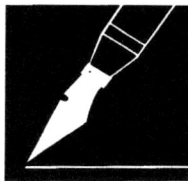

CHAPTER · SEVEN

REEXAMINATIONS

WHAT IS A REASSESSMENT?

Reassessment (Mercy): Evaluation for the purpose of following the progress of a patient under clinical management. The term does not include multiple assessment sessions employed for baseline evaluation and carries the express connotation of assessment performed after the initiation of patient care.

WHAT IS A PERIODIC REASSESSMENT?

Periodic reassessment (Mercy): Evaluation of a patient at intervals of weeks or months for the purpose of assessing the need for continued care, modified care, cessation of care, or referral.

Reevaluations are very important in the management of a patient. You will see less change from visit to visit than you will from month to month. Reevaluations are used to show continued progress and help established the need for continued or future care. It is necessary to evaluate the clinical status and efficacy of care so that decisions about the appropriateness of future care can be made. As a reviewer, I will focus on the reexams more than I do the progress notes. The re-evaluations should be more comprehensive than progress notes and contain more information. Reevaluations include the prior history, current clinical status and interventions utilized so decisions about the necessity and appropriateness of future care can be made.

Progress is defined as a positive change in the patients condition. Progress examinations focus on the same areas that were involved during the initial clinical assessment. Progress examinations also aid in satisfying requirements to third party payers. The frequency of the examinations may vary. If you are seeing someone on a regular basis(at least once per week), it would be wise to do monthly examinations. As a patient gets better or is in a supportive or maintenance mode of care, reevaluations are performed less frequently. Some authors suggest performing reexaminations every 10-12 visits regardless of the stage of treatment. Re-examinations are also the time when you will modify the treatment plan and makes changes according to the patient's progress or lack thereof. This is also where you will show a switch from passive care to active care or a switch to home exercises. Partial reassessment may be done every 2-6 weeks and a complete reassessment is done every 6-12 weeks. The precise frequency may be up to the treating doctor.

ELEMENTS OF A REEVALUATION

1. Patient's self-assessment. (Borg, Oswestry, etc.)

2. Review history. Example: Pain is less frequent than previous exam. What activities and positions can the patient now tolerate that they could not have previously? Has the patient complied with work and/or home care recommendations.

3. New diagnosis or change in diagnosis. (Don't use the word "same.")

4. New treatment plan with the date of the next reevaluation. Has the frequency of visits changed as the patient gets better? Has the number of modalities decreased to correspond with the patient's progress? Has the treatment moved from a passive to active form of treatment?

5. Plan for referrals for testing or evaluations with outside providers.

6. Home care recommendations.

7. Potential discharge date if treatment is nearing an end. Trial of withdrawal? Conditional release?

8. Make sure to list any factors why the patient has not responded to care as expected. If the patient's injury or illness is related to their occupation and they continue to work, this may slow their recovery. Has the patient had any exacerbations?

REEXAMINATION EXAMPLE 1

HISTORY

The patient presents today and states "I have been feeling a lot better." She states there is improvement in both her neck and shoulder pain. She states she has only occasional problems depending on her activities of daily living. She states studying for long periods and carrying her bookbag over her shoulder increases the pain. She denies radiating pain and points to the lower cervical spine and upper trapezius area as the location of the pain. The pain is dull and improved under our care.

She states her mid back has been regressed the last few days. She bent over two days ago and felt an increase in her mid back pain. She relates overall improvement since her first visit. She points to the 5/6 D area as the location of the discomfort. She also states her low back is improved and not giving her any problems. She has been doing her neck exercises at home as directed and using moist heat.

EXAMINATION:

Cervical spine range of motion is within normal limits. There is no pain on resisted cervical spine motion. Upper and lower extremity reflexes are +2/4 bilaterally.

Sensory examination is intact to pain stimulus in the upper and lower extremities. Upper and lower extremity motor function is +5/5 bilaterally. Shoulder Depressor, Spurling's, Allen's, Adson's, Eden's, and Wright's tests are negative bilaterally. Cervical distraction is negative. There are trigger points in the right and left upper traps. Bechterew's, Kemp's, Straight Leg Raising, Nachlas, Femoral Stretch Test, and Sacroiliac Extension tests are negative bilaterally. Lumbar range of motion is within normal limits with no pain. There is joint fixation and tenderness at C5/6 and 5/6D.

ASSESSMENT

Initial diagnosis of acute traumatic cervical acceleration/deceleration syndrome is improved. Cervical, thoracic, and lumbar segmental dysfunctions are improved.

DISCUSSION

Borg pain scale is a 3 today compared to a 6 one month ago. Treatment consisted of an examination, spinal adjustment, and soft tissue technique to the cervical, thoracic, and lumbar spines. She will continue her neck circles at home. We will treat two to three more times and give her a conditional release.

REEXAMINATION EXAMPLE 2

HISTORY

The patient presents and states "up until a couple of days ago I had been feeling relatively better." The patient states his low back is significantly improved over his first visit to this office. He is now able to do all of his activities of daily living. He now has no pain with coughing or sneezing. He states the pain is now mild and intermittent. He has noticed a mild increase in pain the last 1 to 2 days and describes this as a "catch." He is doing his recommended exercises at home as directed and using moist heat at home as well.

EXAMINATION

Lumbar spine range of motion is within normal limits with no pain. There is no pain on resisted range of motion. There is joint fixation and tenderness at L4/5. Lower extremity reflexes are +2/4 bilaterally. Lower extremity motor is +5/5 bilaterally. Lower extremity sensory is intact. Straight Leg Raising, Bechterew's, Femoral Stretch, Nachlas, and Sacroiliac Extension tests are negative bilaterally.

ASSESSMENT

Severe lumbar sprain/strain is resolving.

PLAN

The patient has been instructed to continue the home exercise protocol and return in two weeks. We will consider a conditional release at this time if he continues to be improved.

He has been released to return to his full employment. Today's visit consisted of an examination, spinal adjustment, and myofascial release to the lumbar paraspinal musculature.

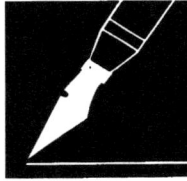

CHAPTER • EIGHT

EXAMINATION

The clinical examination is used to determine a working diagnosis. The examination is used to make appropriate decisions and recommendations for further diagnostic studies and/or treatment. There are several text books available on the topic of examination and orthopedic/neurologic testing. This chapter will not cover examination in great detail but will outline some of the important points and give documentation hints.

COMPONENTS OF AN EXAMINATION

1. **History**

2. **Vital signs:** Gives the examiner a general impression of the patient's overall health status.

   a. *Temperature:* Normal ranges from 96-99.6 in the adult. An increase in the temperature may be due to tissue injury, infection, or burns. A decrease may indicate shock.

   b. *Pulse:* A cardiovascular screening test.
   - Normal rate is 50-100 beats per minute in the adult. Tachycardia (increased pulse) may be due to hyperthyroid or shock. Bradycardia (decreased pulse) may be due a heart blockage or influenza.
   - Normal rhythm is regular
   - Amplitude is the strength of the pulse

   c. *Blood Pressure:* Take in both arms in first visit and when performing George's test.
   - *Normal systolic:* 95-160 mm Hg
   - *Normal diastolic:* 60-90 mm Hg

   d. *Respiration*
   - Average 10-20 breaths per minute

3. **Vertebrobasilar testing**
   a. This testing protocol consists of four parts:
      (1) *History* (Covered previously)
      (2) *Blood Pressure:* Taken in both arms. A 10 mm Hg difference from side to side for the systolic measurement may possibly indicate subclavian artery stenosis or occlusion.
      (3) *Auscultation:* The examiner uses his/her stethoscope to evaluate for a bruit in the subclavian fossa (subclavian artery) and right and left carotid bifurcation (carotid arteries). Remember to have the patient hold their breath for a few seconds when listening to the subclavian fossa. Also, palpate the carotid bifurcation to determine if the pulsation's are normal, feeble, or absent. Some chiropractors decline to do this part of the test because they feel that they aren't well skilled enough with their stethoscope to detect a bruit. (A bruit is not by itself a contraindication)
      (4) *Vertebrobasilar functional maneuvers*
   b. Vertebrobasilar functional maneuvers:
      (1) *George's test:* The patient will rotate his/her head to the right or left as far as possible and then hyperextend the head. This motion decreases the circulation in the atlantoaxial portion of the contralateral vertebral artery. This test is done while the patient is seated. Have the patient count backwards from twenty out loud. Ischemic reactions include vertigo, dizziness, blurred vision, nausea, faintness, and nystagmus.
      (2) Barre-Lieou Sign: The patient is seated and moves head slowly from side to side. Rotation of the head causes compression of the vertebral arteries.
      (3) DeKleyn's test: The patient is supine on the examining table. The head is hyperextended and rotated off of the examination table for 15-45 seconds. The maneuver is repeated on the other side.
      (4) Hallpike maneuver: An enhanced version of the DeKleyn's test. The procedure is similar. The final part allows the patients head to be extremely hyperextended off of the examination table (BE VERY CAREFUL).
   c. Literature review: The best sources for information on VBI and stroke is Dr. Terrett's book "Vertebobasilar Stroke Following Manipulation" published by NCMIC. Dr. Terrett has also published numerous papers on the topic.

4. **General Considerations of Examinations**

   Before performing a examination, the attending doctor must be certain the appropriate information was gathered during the history. Under certain instances (ex. trauma), an x-ray evaluation may be warranted before any orthopedic testing is done. The clinician must assess for contraindications before submitting the patient to provocative tests.

5. **Range of Motion**

   Range of motion is assessed bilaterally and compared to a set of normal values. It is done both actively and passively. Findings are compared to normal values which can vary dramatically, depending on the reference source used. The location, quality, and grade of pain should be noted. An acute injury or severe tissue damage may necessitate the clinician to delay this procedure for several days. The doctor must ask, is the motion consistent with the x-rays, other tests and objective findings? Is motion demonstrated consistent with the nature of injury? Range of motion may vary according to age, sex, and overall flexibility and tone. This test is somewhat dependent on patient compliance and motivation.

Example: Cervical spine flexion is decreased 10 degrees with pain at C5/6; cervical spine extension, right and left lateral flexion, and right and left rotation are within normal limits and there is no pain.

Example: Lumbar spine flexion is decreased 20 degrees with pain at L4/5; lumbar rotation is within normal limits and there is no pain; lumbar spine extension is decreased 15 degrees with pain at L4/5; lumbar spine right and left lateral bending is within normal limits with no pain.

Resisted range of motion is done once active and passive motion has been performed. This is done in flexion, extension, rotation, and lateral bending. This gives the examiner information about the muscle component to an injury. Pain on resisted range of motion indicates a muscular problem. Indicate the resisted motion causing the pain and the location of the pain.

Example: There is pain on resisted cervical spine extension with pain over the lower cervical spine paraspinal musculature; there is no pain on resisted cervical spine flexion, rotation, or lateral bending.

6. **Neurologioc testing**

The neurologic examination is comprised of several different components and is designed to detect neurologic deficits and test the integrity of the nervous system. The neurologic examination locates lesions by testing sensation, muscle strength, deep tendon reflexes, mensuration, and other tests. Neurologic testing includes:

   a. *Mental Examination:* Mental changes include confusion, apathy, depression, anxiety, neurotic behavior, personality disturbances, and mental deterioration. The patients appearance and conduct during the interview includes personal hygiene, appearance, speech, general attitude, posture, and gestures. Family members or friends can be used to obtain general information.

   b. *Cranial Nerves:*

   I. *Olfactory nerve (sensory):* Smell (osmia)—lack of smell is called anosmia. This is tested by having the patient detect different smells one nostril at a time with their eyes closed. Substances that may be used include vanilla, coffee, peppermint, and menthol.

   II. *Optic nerve (sensory):* Vision—confrontation, accommodation, light reflex, consensual reflex. This can be tested by a Snellen eye chart, visual field test, or opthalmoscopic examination.

   III. *Oculomotor:* Motor to the extraocular eye muscles—tested with CN 4 and CN 6. Supplies all of the extrinsic muscles except two: rectus oculi lateralis- abducts eye (CN6) and obliquus oculi superioris-movers eye inferior and laterally (CN4).

IV. *Trochlear:* Tested with abducens (CN6) and oculomotor (CN3). These test motor to the extraocular movements—6 cardinal planes of gaze. Identify paralysis, weakness, nystagmus, conjugate movements (eyes moving together)

V. *Trigeminal (sensory/motor):* Touch, pain, temperature, and motor to the muscles of mastication. The trigeminal nerve has three branches including opthalmic, maxillary, and mandibular. Testing of trigeminal nerve through palpation, i.e., jaw jerk reflex or sensation with a cotton wisp in the three branches. Supplies sensory to most of the face and motor to the muscles of mastication.

VI. *Abducens (motor):* See CN III and CN IV.

VII. *Facial (sensory/motor):* Taste (anterior two thirds of tongue) and facial expression. The sensory portion can be tested by using salt or sugar on the tongue. Closing the eyes or wrinkling the forehead would test the motor portion.

VIII. *Vestibulocochlear (sensory):* Nerve of hearing and equilibrium (balance). This nerve is tested by using a tuning fork. (Weber Rinne)

IX. *Glossopharyngeal (sensory/motor):* Sensory to posterior one third of tongue and motor to swallowing muscles. Taste can be assessed similar to the facial nerve. The gag reflex is tested.

X. *Vagas (motor/sensory):* The patients ability to swallow is tested. The movement of the palate and uvula is determined when the patient says "ah."

XI. *Spinal accessory (motor):* Motor to trapezius and SCM. Tested by having the patient shrug their shoulders against resistance.

XII. *Hypoglossal (motor):* Supplies the muscles of the tongue.

7. **Motor Examination**

a. *Bulk/circumference measurements:* Typically, mensuration in the upper extremity is done just above and below the elbow. In the lower extremity, mensuration is done just above and below the knee. Mensuration is done bilaterally and compared. Atrophy will be indicated by a smaller measurement on the atrophied side.

b. *Tone:* A state of tension in muscles or groups of muscles. Tone may be disturbed in upper motor neuron lesions, lower motor neuron lesions, and sensory disturbances. Decreased muscle tone is called hypotonia while increased muscle tone is called hypertonia. Tone can be diminished or lost when the reflex arc is interrupted. Hypertonic muscles may be classified as spastic or rigid. Rigidity results in diminished passive motion in any direction due to the contraction of flexors and extensors. Spasticity also results in resistance to sudden passive movements. Hypotonic muscles feel soft and flabby.

c. *Muscle strength:* Muscle strength is tested bilaterally and compared. The scale for grading muscle strength is 0-5:

- 5—Normal Full ROM and full resistance against gravity
- 4—Good   Full ROM with some resistance against gravity
- 3—Fair   Full ROM against gravity
- 2—Poor   Full ROM with gravity and resistance eliminated

- 1—Trace   Muscle contraction but no joint movement
- 0—Absent   No evidence of muscle contraction

d. *Myotome:* Individual muscles or groups of muscles supplied by a specific spinal segment. N.R. = Nerve Root.

Myotomal evaluation of the upper extremities include:

- C1-4—Cervical plexus-difficult to isolate
- C1-2—Neck flexion
- C3—Neck lateral flexion
- C4—Shoulder elevation and diaphragm
- C5—Arm abduction-deltoid
- C6—Wrist extensors, biceps
- C7—Wrist flexors, triceps
- C8—Finger flexors (grip)
- T1—Includes finger abductors and adductors

Myotomal evaluation of the lower extremities includes:

- L 4 N.R. (L3-4 disc): Quadriceps
- L5 N.R. (L4-5 disc): Dorsiflexion of great toe and foot; difficulty walking on heels; foot drop may occur.
- S1 N.R. (L5-S1 disc): Plantar flexion of foot and great toe; difficulty walking on toes; gluteus maximus

    Example: Upper extremity motor function is +5/5 bilaterally.

    Example: Biceps is +4/5 right and +5/5 left; triceps, deltoid, and grip are +5/5 bilaterally.

8. **Reflexes:** Involuntary motor responses to sensory stimuli. These may be divided into superficial, muscle stretch, and pathological reflexes. Muscle stretch reflexes are present in a normal person and can be produced by a sudden stretch of the muscle. Examples of muscle stretch reflexes include the biceps and triceps and they are tested bilaterally. Superficial reflexes are also present under normal circumstances and include the corneal, gag, and superficial abdominal.

   a. *Muscle stretch reflexes/Deep tendon reflexes:* Grading these reflexes is done by using the following scale:

   0—Absent

   1—Hypoactive

   2—Normal

   3—Hyperactive

   4—Hyperactive with clonus

   Example: Upper extremity reflexes are +2/4 bilaterally.

   Example: Triceps is +1/4 right and +2/4 left; biceps and brachioradialis are +2/4 bilaterally.

9. **Sensory Function**

Dermatomes are areas of skin supplied by a single spinal segment. These areas vary according to the reference and are not totally specific. They may give the examiner information regarding an involved spinal segment. The area supplied may also be supplied by the nerve root above and/or below. This is why they are not totally specific.

Typically dermatomes are tested with a pinwheel for pain sensation or a cotton swab for light touch. The patient is asked if they have an increase, decrease, altered, or absent sensation. Findings are indicated as follows:

- Hyperasthetic = Increased sensation
- Hypoasethic = Decreased sensation
- Dysthetic = Altered sensation
- Anesthesia = Absent

Example: There is a decrease in sensation to pain stimulus in the C5 dermatome on the right. All other upper extremity dermatomes show no abnormalities.

10. **Orthopedic Tests**

These tests may vary somewhat depending on the text that is being used. They are designed to mimic movements that cause pain, thereby reproducing the pain. Contraindications should be assessed before performing an orthopedic examination. Also, certain tests are not to be done in acute or severe conditions.

Selected Orthopedic Tests

a. *Libman's Test:* A general test for pain threshold. The examiner places pressure on the mastoid process. Someone with a low pain threshold will jump when a slight amount of pressure is applied.

b. *Lhermitte's Sign:* Present when the patient experiences a shock-like sensation when they flex their cervical spine. Indicative of a cord lesion such as multiple sclerosis, or degeneration of the posterior columns.

c. *Mankopf's:* A test for true pain. The examiner first determines the patient's pulse. The examiner then puts pressure on the area of alleged pain and again measures the pulse with the pressure being applied. True pain will increase the pulse at least ten beats per minute.

d. *O'Donaghue's:* This test differentiates between sprain and strain. Pain on passive motion is indicative joint/ligament pain. Pain on resisted motion is indicative of muscle injury.

e. *Rust signs:* Indicates possible severe cervical trauma. The patient holds their head up with their hands.

f. *Valsalva's Maneuver:* The patient is asked to strain down as if they were going to have a bowel movement. Increased pain resulting from increased intrathecal pressure is usually indicative of a space occupying lesion (HNP, tumor, osteophytes). A true positive tests has a radicular pain referral.

g. *Triad of DeJerine:* Coughing, sneezing, or straining on defecation causes aggravation of radicular symptoms.

h. *Foraminal Compression Tests:* These tests induce movements closing the intervertebral foramen in the cervical spine. A positive test is indicated by radicular pain and the doctor must then assess nerve root function. There are several different variations to this test and they differ slightly depending on the reference text used.

i. *Straight Leg Raising Test (SLR):* The patient lies supine with the legs extended. The examiner places one hand under the heel and the other hand on the knee. The examiner then raises the affected leg. This test is positive if the pain extends from the back, down the leg along the sciatic nerve distribution. Central protrusions of an intervertebral disc cause pain in the back. Intermediate protrusions cause low back and lower limb pain. Lateral protrusions will cause primarily posterior leg pain. The SLR will cause traction on the sciatic nerve, lumbosacral nerve roots, and dura mater.

After pain is produced with this test, the leg is lowered just below the point where pain is produced. The examiner then dorsiflexes the foot (Braggard's) and can also have the patient flex his/her neck (Hyndman's sign). Pain that is increased with foot dorsiflexion, neck flexion, or both results from stretching of the dura mater of the spinal cord. Pain that does not increase with neck flexion or foot dorsiflexion may indicate tight hamstrings, lumbosacral, or sacroiliac involvement.

Unilateral SLR is full at 60-70 degrees. Pain after 60-70 degrees is probably due to sacroiliac involvement. The degree at which pain is produced is always recorded.

Examples: Straight Leg Raising Test is positive on the right at 40 degrees with pain in the lower lumbar spine and radiating down the posterior aspect of the right leg to the knee. Braggard's test is positive on the right with dorsiflexion of the foot increasing pain. Neck flexion also results in an increase in lumbar spine and radicular pain.

j. *Bechterew's Sitting Test:* The patient is seated and attempts to extend each leg one at a time. Then attempts to extend both legs. The test is positive if backache or sciatic pain is increased or the patient is unable to do the maneuver. With disc involvement, extending both legs will usually increase spinal and sciatic discomfort. A positive test indicates sciatica, disc involvement, adhesions, spasm, or subluxation.

k. *Braggard's Sign:* If the Straight Leg Raising test is positive, the leg is lowered just below the level of discomfort and the foot is sharply dorsiflexed. The sign is present if the pain is increased. The test indicates nerve root inflammation. If the test does not increase the pain, then the positive SLR may indicate a problem in the hamstring area or in the lumbosacral or sacroiliac joints.

l. *Cox Sign:* This occurs during SLR when the pelvis rises from the table instead of the hip flexing. Cox signs is present when patients have a prolapse of the nucleus into the IVF.

m. *Fajersztajn's Test:* SLR and dorsiflexion of the foot are performed on the asymptomatic side of a sciatic patient. The sign is present when the test causes pain on the symptomatic side. This test indicates nerve root involvement.

n. *Kemp's Test:* The patient is seated or standing with their arms crossed. The patient is then rotated and extended without moving their pelvis. A positive test produces pain in a radicular pattern indicating nerve root compression. Localized pain is not a true positive test but this suggests facet inflammation.

o. *Nachlas Test:* The patient is prone and the knee is passively flexed. Pain in the low back or lower extremity is positive and indicates a sacroiliac or lumbosacral disorder.

p. *Gaenslen's Test:* The patient is lying supine. The examiner flexes the knee and thigh of the unaffected leg to the abdomen. The patient is brought to the end of the table and the examiner slowly extends the affected thigh. The test is positive for pain in the sacroiliac area or referred down the thigh. The test is usually contraindicated in geriatrics. Sacroiliac involvement produces local pain over the joint, or pain that is referred to the groin on the same side, the posterior thigh on the same side, and down the leg, which is less often. Pain is often increased by lying on the affected side.

q. *Well Leg Raising Test:* This test is the same as the straight leg raising test but is performed on the unaffected leg. The patient is supine and the examiner places one hand under the heel and the other hand on the knees. This test is positive when it produces pain in the back and down the affected leg. This test is followed by the Fajersztajn's Test.

11. **Chiropractic Analysis:** This is what separates chiropractic from other health care professions. These procedures are used to detect the vertebral subluxation complex. These procedures include:

a. Visualization
   - Posture
   - Inspection

b. Instrumentation

c. Leg checks

d. Static palpation (edema, muscle tone, spasm, etc.)

e. Motion palpation-looking for joint fixation
   - Fixation = loss of joint motion
   - Indicators of fixation include: decreased ROM, loss of joint play, crepitance (noise in joint) and stuttering (catches in joint).

f. X-ray analysis

12. **Regional Examinations:** The following is an overview of a general examination for certain regions. The complexity of the examination is in direct proportion to the patients history, mechanism of injury, prior history, and other historical information.

a. Cervical Spine Examination

   The typical cervical spine examination includes the following:
   - Vital Signs
   - Range of motion
   - Resisted range of motion
   - Reflex testing

- Motor testing
- Sensory testing
- Vertebrobasilar Testing
- O'Donoghue's maneuver
- Foraminal Compression testing
- Shoulder Depressor
- Other tests may include: Soto Hall, Allen's, Eden's, Wright's, Adson's, and Cervical Distraction.
- Chiropractic Analysis

b. Lumbosacral Examination
- Range of motion
- Resisted range of motion
- Reflex testing
- Motor testing
- Sensory testing
- Chiropractic Analysis
- Valsalva's Maneuver
- Kemp's Test
- Bechterew's Test
- Straight Leg Raising Test/Braggard's
- Well Leg raising Test/Fajersztajn's
- Gaenslen's Test
- Sacroiliac Extension Test
- Fabere Patrick
- Hibbs

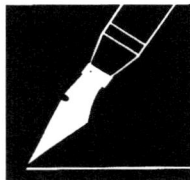

CHAPTER • NINE

LITERATURE REVIEW

Carpal Tunnel Syndrome

A. *Definition:* Compression of the median nerve in the carpal tunnel between the transverse carpal ligament and the bones of the wrist and hand. The median nerve supplies sensation to the thumb, first and second finger, and half of your ring finger.

B. *Signs and Symptoms:*
- Numbness or tingling over the radial aspect of the hand.
- Pain in the wrist, hand, or arm. Pain may radiate as far as the shoulder.
- Weakness or atrophy in muscles of the hand supplied by the median nerve.
- Repetitive use increases sensory symptoms.
- The symptoms are most apparent at night.
- Lack of coordination of the hands.
- Family history

C. *High Risk Jobs:*
- Data entry
- Meat packing
- Electronics assemblers
- Waiter/Waitress
- Beauticians
- Carpenters
- Construction workers
- Garment workers
- Frozen food processors
- Pregnancy
- Jobs where the hands are in awkward positions
- Jobs that use vibrating hand tools.

D. *Etiology:*
- Forceful frequent gripping
- Injury such as following a wrist fracture.
- Occupations causing microtrauma
- Frequent positions of wrist flexion or extension
- "double crush"

E. *Non-Work Related Risk Factors:*
- Diabetes and hypothyroidism.
- Sex. Females are affected three times more than men.
- Age. More common in people between 30 and 50 years of age.
- Smoking. CTS is more common in smokers.
- Peripheral neuropathies such as those induced by alcoholism or chemotherapy.
- Carpal tunnel syndrome on the other side
- Pregnancy. This is due to increased swelling in the carpal tunnel.

F. *Clinical Presentation:*
- Symptom picture suggestive of CTS. Proximal arm symptoms may be present.
- Loss of grip strength. Thenar atrophy is a late feature.
- Decreased sensation over the course of the median nerve. Patients presenting in the early stages may have no sensory loss.
- Positive provocative tests such as Tinel, Phalen, LeBan, and tourniquet tests.
- Special testing procedures (EMG/NCV, MRI).
- According to NIOSH, a diagnosis of CTS should include objective findings consistent with CTS, either:
   - one or more of the following physical findings: Tinel sign, Phalen sign or decreased or absent sensation to pin prick in the median nerve distribution of the hand, or
   - electrodiagnostic findings of median nerve dysfunction across the carpal tunnel.

G. *Electrodiagnostic testing:*
- Tests such as the EMG and NCV are approximately 90% accurate in detecting carpal tunnel syndrome. Carpal tunnel syndrome may still be present in the absence of a positive test.

H. *Orthopedic testing:*
- *Tinel's sign:* Percussion of the median nerve at the wrist. A positive test reproduces paresthesia in the distribution of the median nerve. False positives may range from (6-45%) depending on the reference.
- *Phalen's sign:* The patient hold the hands in flexion and forearms vertically for about one minute. Positive findings are numbness or paresthesia in the distribution of the median nerve.

- *Tourniquet test:* Occlusion of forearm blood flow. Patients with CTS develop their symptoms of hand paresthesias or sensory loss in a median distribution.

I.   *Other Contributory factors:*
- Knitting
- Musical instruments
- Hobbies-wood working, gardening.
- Birth control pills
- Incorrect sleeping position
- Sitting on hands

J.   *Treatment:*
1. Rest- Work and home modifications.
2. Splinting
3. Anti-inflammatory medication
4. Corticosteroid injections
5. Surgery
6. Exercises
7. Manipulation and modalities
8. Nutritional supplementation

The complete evaluation of a patient with upper extremity complaints would include and examination of the cervical spine, shoulder, and elbow. The term "double crush" was first used by Upton and McComas. This refers to proximal compression on a nerve causing distal symptoms. This can be done by mechanical pressure and metabolic conditions. Differential diagnosis with CTS includes: rheumatoid arthritis, degenerative arthritis, diabetes mellitus, oral contraceptive, thyroid, gout, and obesity.

THORACIC OUTLET SYNDROME

A.   *Definition:* This is a condition where symptoms are produced by compression of nerve or blood vessels or both because of inadequate passageway between the base of the neck and the axilla. Compression may occur at the scalene muscles, under the clavicle, or through the axilla.

B.   *Signs and Symptoms:* Neck, shoulder, arm pain/numbness; impaired circulation. Symptoms reproduced when arm is above the shoulder. Weakness, especially when the arm is above the head. Cold sensitivity, pallor, swelling and temperature aberrations are less common and are thought to be secondary to vascular compression.

C.   *Etiology:*
  • Violent injury such as with a car accident (shoulder harness)
  • Cervical rib
  • Using heavy pocketbooks and backpacks
  • Sleeping with the arm above the head
  • Working with the arm over the head for long periods
  • Hypertrophy of pectoralis muscle from weightlifting

D.   *Examination:*
  • Since this condition can mimic cervical disc problems and CTS, these must be checked.
  • EMG and SSEP can be used to help detect TOS.
  • Orthopedic examinations:

   1.   *Allen's*—Tests the patency of the radial and ulnar arteries. A positive test is lack of blood return. This could mean possible arterial blockage and a vascular consultation may be indicated.

   2.   *Adson's test*—The patient is seated. The examiner palpates the radial pulse and asks the patient to rotate their head and slightly extend it while the examiner externally rotates the shoulder. This disappearance of a pulse is a positive test indicating scalenus anticus or cervical rib TOS. The scalene muscles originate from the TVPs of the cervical vertebrae and insert on the first and second ribs. A foramen admits the subclavian artery and the brachial plexus.

   3.   *Eden's/Costoclavicular test*—The patient is seated. The examiner palpates the radial pulse while drawing the patients shoulder down and into extension. The patient then flexes the chin to the chest. The test is positive when the pulse is absent. This indicates compression of the neurovascular bundle as it enters the axilla beneath the clavicle and on top of the first rib.

   4.   *Wright's test/Hyperabduction maneuver*—The patient is seated. The examiner abducts the patients arm to 180 degrees while palpating the radial pulse. The degree at which the pulse disappears is noted and compared to the unaffected side. Paresthesia and radicular symptoms are noted when they are reproduced.

E.   *Treatment:*
  • Work and home modifications: Sleep instructions, avoid heavy lifting, working with arms abducted for long periods, carrying shoulder bags.
  • Shoulder shrug exercises
  • Physical therapy modalities
  • Chiropractic adjustments
  • Surgery

F.   *Literature:*
   1.   "Thoracic Outlet Syndrome in Cervical Strain Injury" by T. Capistrant M.D., *Minnesota Medicine*, Vol. 69, January 1986. Thoracic outlet syndrome is associated with cervical strain injuries, especially

flexion/extension whiplash injuries commonly caused by rear-end collisions. This study found that thoracic outlet developed in 36% of the cases of cervical strain injuries. Thoracic outlet may initially be overshadowed by other complaints such as neck pain or headaches that are common in whiplash patients.

2. "The T 4 Syndrome" by Defranca and Levine, *JMPT*, Vol. 18, #1, 1995. This article is very important in the treatment of cervical, thoracic, and upper extremity complaints. Clinical features of the T4 syndrome include paresthesia, numbness, or upper extremity pains associated with or without headache and upper back stiffness. There are no hard neurological signs. The symptoms stem from joint dysfunction in the upper thoracic spine, particularly the T4 segment. A non-traumatic onset is common and the peculiar glove-like distribution of hand and forearm pain can often lead to a mistaken diagnosis, including psychogenesis. Any segment from T2-7 can be involved but T4 is the most common. Neurovascular signs are not a feature. Women are more affected than males by a ratio of 4:1. The most common age group is 30-50. Postural strain due to prolonged sitting is thought to be a contributing factor. Sustained reaching and pulling is contributory. Upper extremity symptoms are glove-like, involve the hand, forearm or entire upper extremity and are usually bilaterally. Nocturnal occurrence of upper extremity symptoms are characteristic with the patient usually awoken with paresthesia of hands or arms either in the middle of the night or in the morning. Getting up or shaking the hands and arms usually alleviates the symptoms. Symptoms typically start as a nuisance and get worse over time. Differential diagnosis includes carpal tunnel syndrome, thoracic outlet syndrome, cervical disc herniation, myofascial pain syndrome, and psychogenic pain. Examination findings: Cervical and thoracic ROM WNL; neurologics negative;vascular tests negative; stiff mid and upper back; head forward posture (tight pectorals); x-ray is negative; trigger points in the pectoralis major and mid traps. Treatment consists of flexion exercises, postural advice, and adjustments.

COMPLICATING FACTORS

The following three tables indicate conditions or factors that may complicate or prolong recovery of musculoskeletal disorders. Look at these three lists carefully and see how they compare.

(From C. Liebenson, *Rehabilitation of the Spine: A Practitioner's Manual.* Williams & Wilkins, 1996.)

HISTORY/CONSULTATION

• Previous history of low back pain

• More than four episodes

• Total work loss in past 12 months

• Heavy smoking

• Personal problems: alcohol, marital, financial

- Adversarial medicolegal problems
- Longer than one week of symptoms before presenting to doctor
- Low education attainment
- Heavy physical occupation

QUESTIONNAIRES/PAIN DRAWINGS OR SCALES

- Radiating leg pain
- Severe pain intensity
- Low job satisfaction
- Psychological distress and depressive symptoms

EXAMINATION

- Pre-existing structural pathology or skeletal anomaly (i.e. spondylolisthesis) directly related to new injury or condition
- Reduced straight leg raising
- Signs of nerve root involvement
- Reduced trunk strength and endurance
- Poor physical fitness (aerobic capacity)
- Disproportionate illness behavior (Waddell's signs)

RISK FACTORS CHRONICITY (BRITISH GUIDELINES FOR BACK PAIN)

(From G. Waddell, *The Low Back Pain Guidelines* [British]. Clinical Standards Advisory Group: Back Pain, London, HMSO, 1994.)

- Previous history of low back pain
- Total work loss (because of low back pain) in past 12 months
- Radiating leg pain
- Reduced straight leg raising
- Signs of nerve root involvement
- Reduced trunk strength and endurance
- Poor physical fitness
- Self-rated poor health
- Heavy smoking
- Psychological distress and depressive symptoms
- Disproportionate illness behavior
- Low job satisfaction
- Personal problems-alcohol, marital, financial
- Adversarial medicolegal proceedings

COMMON FACTORS POTENTIALLY COMPLICATING CAD TRAUMA MANAGEMENT

(From: A. Croft, S. Foreman, *Whiplash Injuries: The Acceleration/Deceleration Syndrome*, Williams and Wilkins, 1996)

1. Advanced age
2. Metabolic disorders
3. Congenital anomalies of the spine
4. Developmental anomalies of the spine
5. Degenerative disc disease
6. Disc protrusions (HNP)
7. Spondylosis
8. Facet arthrosis
9. Rheumatoid arthritis or other arthritides affecting the spine
10. Ankylosing spondylitis or other spondyloarthropathy
11. Scoliosis
12. Prior cervical spine surgery
13. Prior lumbar spine surgery
14. Prior vertebral fracture
15. Osteoporosis
16. Paget's disease or other disease of bone
17. Spinal stenosis or foraminal stenosis
18 Paraplegia or quadriplegia
19. Prior spinal surgery

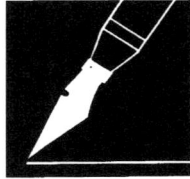

CHAPTER • TEN

UTILIZATION GUIDELINES

This chapter contains several different sets of guidelines. They are not to be used as an absolute cutoff point for any specific case. Each case is different with its own set of clinical findings, diagnosis, and complicating factors and should be viewed for its own merits. These guidelines are intended to be flexible. Many factors must be considered in determining clinical or medical necessity. These guidelines are to assist the practitioner in helping to determine when additional information may be needed. Exacerbations and reinjuries may prolong recovery. These guidelines are not standards of care but serve as a general guide.

The current guidelines are based on the current scientific literature and practice trends and may change. Patients may respond differently and at a rate slower than anticipated. The need for proper documentation to allow for good communication between the doctor and insurance company cannot be overstated.

These guidelines represent reasonable and appropriate treatment for optimum recovery. Each case has its own specific parameters and may require less or more treatment depending on the clinical circumstances. Treatment should be based on patient need and good sound professional judgment but some atypical cases may fall outside these guidelines.

Early return to activity and recognizing the factors that cause chronicity will help reduce disability and chronicity. The warning signs of chronicity include: anxiety or depression, family turmoil, somatic complaints that remain static longer than two to three weeks, functional or emotional disability and drug dependence. Long term outcome and prognosis decreases with an increase in time and the patient should be reevaluated every 2-4 weeks.

DEFINITIONS

Adequate Trial of Treatment/Care (Mercy): A course of two weeks each of two different types of manual procedures (four weeks total), after which, in the absence of documented improvement, manual procedures are no longer indicated.

Complicated case (Mercy): A case where the patient, because of one or more identifiable factors, exhibits regression or retarded recovery in comparison with expectations from the natural history.

Uncomplicated case (Mercy): A case where the patient exhibits progressive recovery from illness or injury at a rate greater than, or equal to, the expectation from the natural history.

Natural history (Mercy): The anticipated clinical course of recovery for uncomplicated disorders either without treatment/care or with conservative treatment/care.

Passive care (Mercy): Application of treatment/care modalities by the care-giver to a patient, who "passively" receives care.

Active care (Mercy): Modes of treatment/care requiring "active" involvement, participation, and responsibility on the part of the patient.

Maintenance/Preventive Care (Mercy): Appropriate professionally acceptable treatment usually for a chronic condition or after completion of therapeutic or supportive care, directed at a symptomatically stationary condition with anticipation of maintaining optimal body function, and usually provided on some routine or regular basis. Continued treatment after a patient has reached MMI, resolution, and/or stabilization of a condition would constitute maintenance type care in nature.

Supportive care (Mercy): Treatment/care for patients having reached MMI, in whom periodic trials of withdrawal from care fail to sustain previous therapeutic gains that would otherwise progressively deteriorate. Supportive care follows appropriate application of active and passive care including lifestyle modifications. It is appropriate when rehabilitative and/or functional restorative and alternative care options, including home-based self-care and lifestyle modifications, have been considered and attempted. Supportive care may be inappropriate when it interferes with other appropriate primary care, or when the risk of supportive care outweighs its benefits, i.e., physician dependence, somatization, illness behavior, and secondary gain.

Therapeutic Necessity: Exists in the presence of an impairment evidenced by recognized signs and symptoms, and likely to respond favorably to the treatment/care planned.

Treatment Plan (Mercy): A written description of intended therapeutic actions divided according to relevant treatment/care goals and prognosis.

Treatment/Care Dynamics-Manual Procedures (Mercy):

1. Threshold: The minimum rate and magnitude of joint load needed to bring about change.
2. Dosage: The frequency of care necessary and sufficient to maintain effects while healing occurs.
3. Duration: The minimum treatment/care interval to obtain a stable response.

4. Combination: The potentiation or competition of response by simultaneous treatment/care applications.

MERCY GUIDELINES
(Material reprinted with permission)
Stages of Treatment/Care: (sequential or concurrent)

1. Acute interventions: Initial therapeutic interventions to assist and promote anatomical rest, reduce muscle spasm and inflammatory reaction, and alleviate pain.

2. Remobilization: Continuing intervention to increase the pain free ranges of motion and to minimize deconditioning.

3. Efforts to restore strength and endurance in the pain free range, and increase physical work capacity. Rehabilitation is treatment/care applied for more chronic or complex problems in patients with impaired capabilities. It may be used sequentially or concomitantly with other care depending on the specific characteristics of the problem.

4. Lifestyle Adaptations: Adaptations of lifestyle necessary to modify social and recreational activity, diminish work environment risk factors, and adapt to psychological elements affecting, or altered by, the disorder.

Short- and Long-Range Treatment Planning:

1. Preconsultation duration of symptoms. Pain less than eight days = no anticipated delay in recovery. Pain more than 8 days = Recovery may take 1.5 times longer.

2. Typical severity of symptoms. Mild pain = No anticipated delay in recovery. Severe pain = recovery may take up to two times longer.

3. Number of Previous episodes. 0-3 episodes = No anticipated delay in recovery. 4-7 episodes = recovery may take up to two times longer.

4. Injury superimposed on preexisting conditions. Skeletal anomaly or structural pathology may increase recovery two times longer.

TREATMENT/CARE FREQUENCY

Specific recommendations related to acute, subacute and chronic presentations are given below. In general, more aggressive in-office interventions (3-5 sessions per week for 1-2 weeks) may be necessary early. Progressively declining frequency is expected to discharge of the patient, or conversion to elective care.

FAILURE TO MEET TREATMENT/CARE OBJECTIVES

1. Acute Disorders: After a maximum of two trial therapy series of manual procedures lasting up to two weeks each(four weeks total) without significant documented improvement, manual procedures may no longer be appropriate and alternative care should be considered.

2. Unresponsive Acute, Subacute, or Chronic Disorders: Repeated use of passive treatment/care normally designed to manage acute conditions should be avoided as it tends to promote physician dependence and chronicity.

3. Systematic interview of the patient and the immediate family should be carried out in search for complicating or extenuating factors responsible for prolonged recovery.

4. Specific treatment/care goals should be written to address each issue.

5. Continued failure should result in patient discharge as inappropriate for chiropractic care, or having achieved maximum therapeutic benefit.

UNCOMPLICATED CASE: (ACUTE EPISODE)

1. *Symptom response:* Significant improvement within 10-14 days; 3-5 treatments per week.

2. *Activities of Daily Living (ADL):* The promotion of rest, elevation, and remobilization, as needed, are expected to improve ADL followed by a favorable response in symptoms.

3. *Return to PreEpisode Status:* six to eight weeks; up to three treatments per week

4. *Supportive Care:* Inappropriate

COMPLICATED CASES

1. *Signs of Chronicity:* All episodes of symptoms that remain unchanged for two to three weeks should be evaluated for risk factors of pending chronicity. Patients at risk for becoming chronic should have treatment plans altered to de-emphasize passive care and refocus on active care approaches.

2. *Subacute Episode*
   a. *Symptom Response:* Symptoms have been prolonged beyond six weeks, and passive care in this phase is as necessary, not generally to exceed two treatments per week, to avoid promoting chronicity or physician dependence.
   b. *Activities of Daily Living (ADL):* Management emphasis shifts to active care, dissuasion of pain behavior, patient education, flexibility and stabilization exercises. Rehabilitation may be appropriate.
   c. *Return to Preepisode status:* 6-16 weeks (12-32 office visits)
   d. *Supportive care:* Inappropriate

3. *Chronic Episode*
   a. *Symptom response:* Symptoms have been prolonged beyond 16 weeks. Use of passive care beyond 16 weeks is for exacerbation only.
   b. *Activities of Daily Living (ADL):* Supervised rehabilitation and life style changes are appropriate.
   c. *Return to Preinjury status:* May not return. Maximum therapeutic benefit should be considered.
   d. *Supportive care:* Supportive care using passive therapy may be necessary if repeated efforts to withdraw treatment/care result in significant deterioration of clinical status.

NORTH AMERICAN SPINE SOCIETY

These guidelines were developed in 1993 and include common therapeutic procedure used in the treatment of lumbosacral disorders. The natural history of most lumbar spine pain syndromes is 90-120 days(3-4 months) following the initial onset of pain.

MANUAL THERAPY

- Treatment frequency: 2-5 supervised treatments per week for the first two weeks, decreasing to 1-2 treatments per week

- Optimum treatment duration: 1 month

- Maximum treatment duration: 2-4 months

Other excerpts from the North American Spine Society Guidelines are found in Chapter 13.

OKLAHOMA WORKERS' COMPENSATION LOW BACK PAIN GUIDELINES
(Sept. 8, 1995)

The development of these guidelines included the North American Spine Society, Mercy, and AHCPR Guidelines. The Oklahoma guideline stresses the importance of re-evaluating the patient every two to four weeks to modify treatment. History, physical examination, x-ray, and laboratory tests were all used for the diagnosis of a work-related low back complaint. Excerpts include:

Manipulation

Aggressive in-office intervention (3-5 sessions per week for 1-2 weeks) may be necessary early to stabilized the patients condition. The typical range of visits is 5-18 with a progressively declining frequency until the patient is discharged. Significant improvement within 10-14 days should be seen. Additional excerpts are found in chapter 13.

FLORIDA GUIDELINES

Duration of Care

Initial/Therapeutic—14-45 days as necessitated by subjective/ objective findings and documentation.

Reconstructive—45-180 days as necessitated by subjective/objective findings and documentation.

Supportive—As necessitated by subjective/ objective findings and documentation.

ACUTE LOW BACK PROBLEMS IN ADULTS: ASSESSMENT AND TREATMENT

The following pages contain the tables and algorithms from this guideline. This guideline is exclusively for acute low back pain in adults. This was constructed by a multidisciplinary panel of experts who did an extensive review of the literature. The history portion of this guideline was covered previously in Chapter 5.

AHCPR Guideline 14
Acute Low Back Problems in Adults: Assessment and Treatment

Algorithm 1   Initial evaluation of acute low back problem

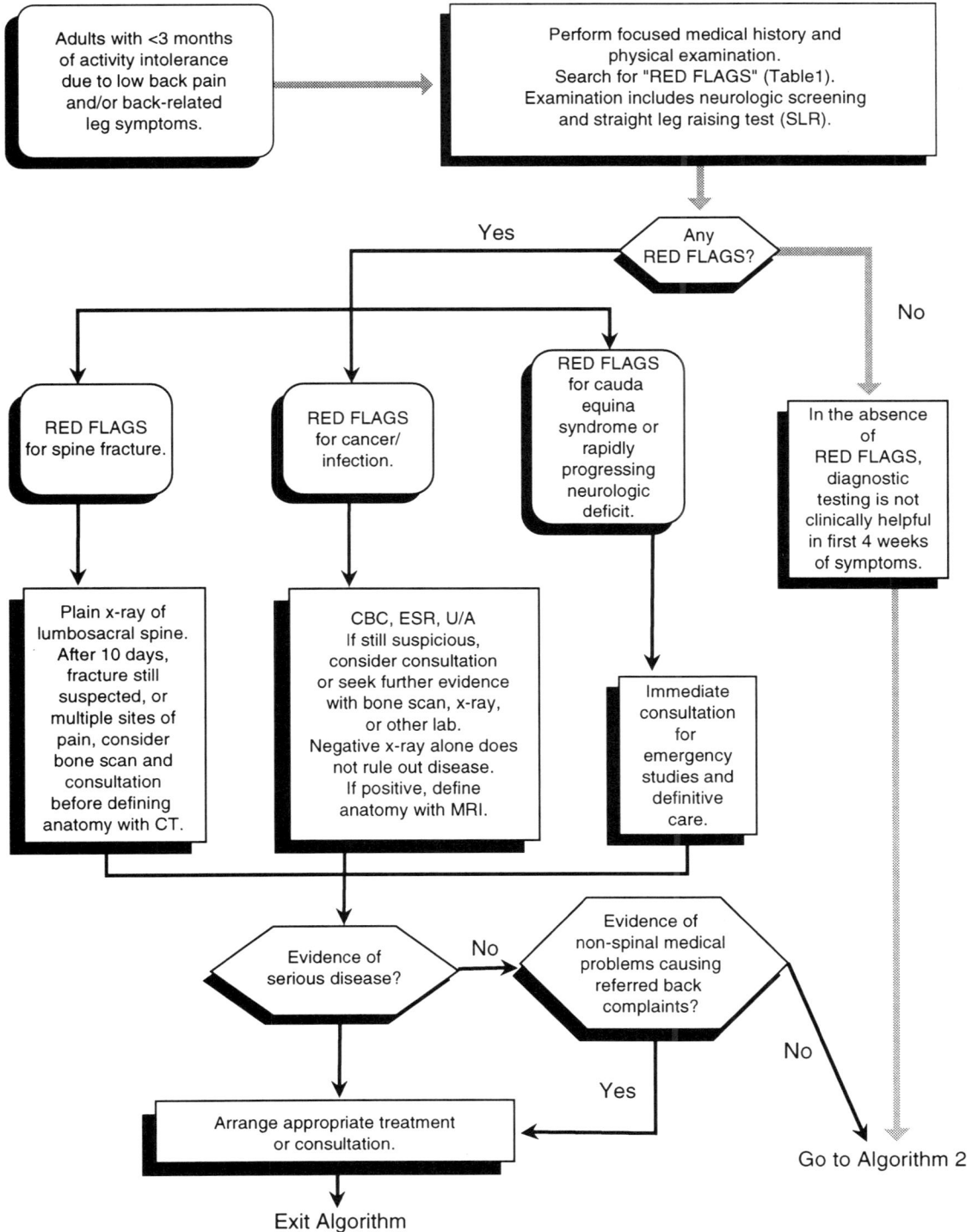

Algorithm 2   Treatment of acute low back problem on initial and followup visits

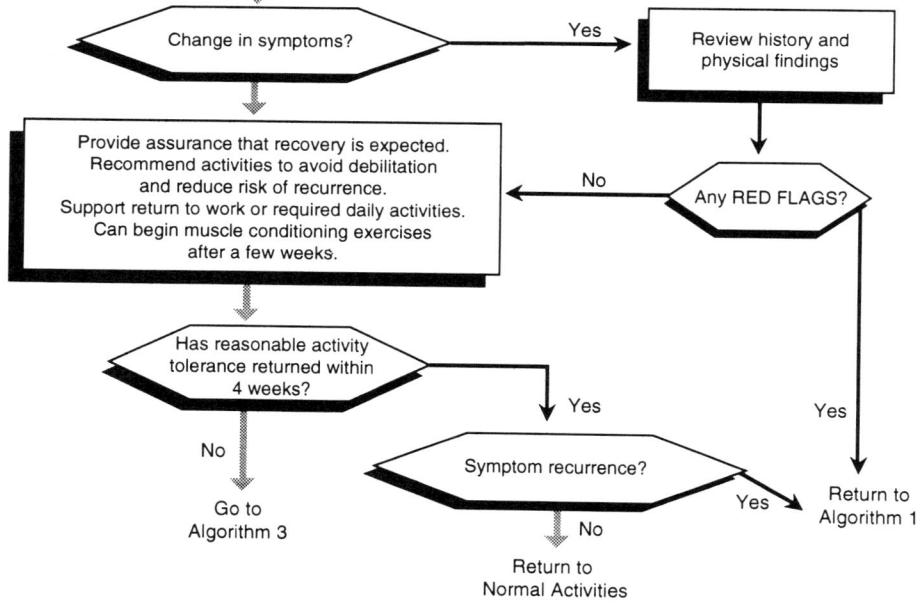

Initial visit

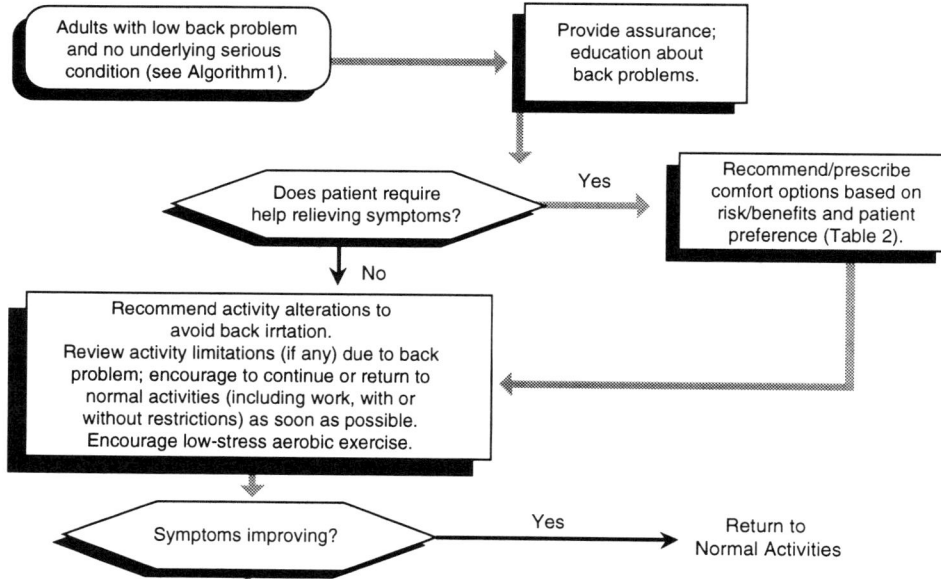

Adults with low back problem and no underlying serious condition (see Algorithm1).

Provide assurance; education about back problems.

Does patient require help relieving symptoms?

Yes

Recommend/prescribe comfort options based on risk/benefits and patient preference (Table 2).

No

Recommend activity alterations to avoid back irrtation.
Review activity limitations (if any) due to back problem; encourage to continue or return to normal activities (including work, with or without restrictions) as soon as possible.
Encourage low-stress aerobic exercise.

Symptoms improving?

Yes

Return to Normal Activities

Followup visits

Change in symptoms?

Yes

Review history and physical findings

Provide assurance that recovery is expected.
Recommend activities to avoid debilitation and reduce risk of recurrence.
Support return to work or required daily activities.
Can begin muscle conditioning exercises after a few weeks.

No

Any RED FLAGS?

Yes

Has reasonable activity tolerance returned within 4 weeks?

No

Go to Algorithm 3

Yes

Symptom recurrence?

Yes

Return to Algorithm 1

No

Return to Normal Activities

Table 1. Red flags for potentially serious conditions		
Possible fracture	Possible tumor or infection	Possible cauda equina syndrome
From medical history		
Major trauma, such as vehicle accident or fall from height. Minor trauma or even strenuous lifting (in older potentially osteoporotic patient)	Age over 50 or under 20. History of cancer. Constitutional symptoms, such as recent fever or chills or unexplained weight loss. Risk factors for spinal infection: recent bacterial infection (e.g., uninary tract infection); IV drug abuse; or immune suppression (from steroids, transplant, or HIV). Pain that worsens when supine; severe nighttime pain.	Saddle anesthesia. Recent onset of bladder dysfunction, such as urinary retention, increased frequency, or overflow incontinence. Severe or progressive neurologic deficit in the lower extremity.
From physical examination		
		Unexpected laxity of the anal sphincter. Perianal/perineal sensory loss. Major motor weakness: quadriceps (knee extension weakness); ankle plantar flexors, evertors, and dorsiflexors (foot drop).

Table 2. Symptom control methods		
Recommended		
Nonprescription analgesics		
Acetaminophen (safest) NSAIDs (Aspirin,[1] Ibuprofen[1])		
Prescribed pharmeaceutical methods	**Prescribed physical methods**	
Nonspecific low back symptoms and / or sciatica	**Nonspecific low back symptoms**	**Sciatica**
Other NSAIDs[1]	Manipulation (in place of medication or a shorter trial if combined with NSAIDs)	
Options		
Nonspecific low back symptoms and / or sciatica	**Nonspecific low back symptoms**	**Sciatica**
Muscle relaxants [2,3,4] Opioids [2,3,4]	Physical agents and modalities [2] (heat or cold modalities for home programs only) Shoe insoles [2]	Manipulation (in place of medication or a shorter trial if combined with NSAIDs) Physical agents and modalities [2] (heat or cold modalities for home programs only) Few days rest [4] Shoe insoles [2]

[1] Aspirin and other NSAIDs are not recommended for use in combination with one another due to the
risk of GI complications.
[2] Equivocal efficacy.
[3] Significant potential for producing drowsiness and debilitation; potential for dependency.
[4] Short course (few days only) for severe symptoms.

Algorithm 3   Evaluation of slow - to - recover patient (symptoms> 4 weeks)

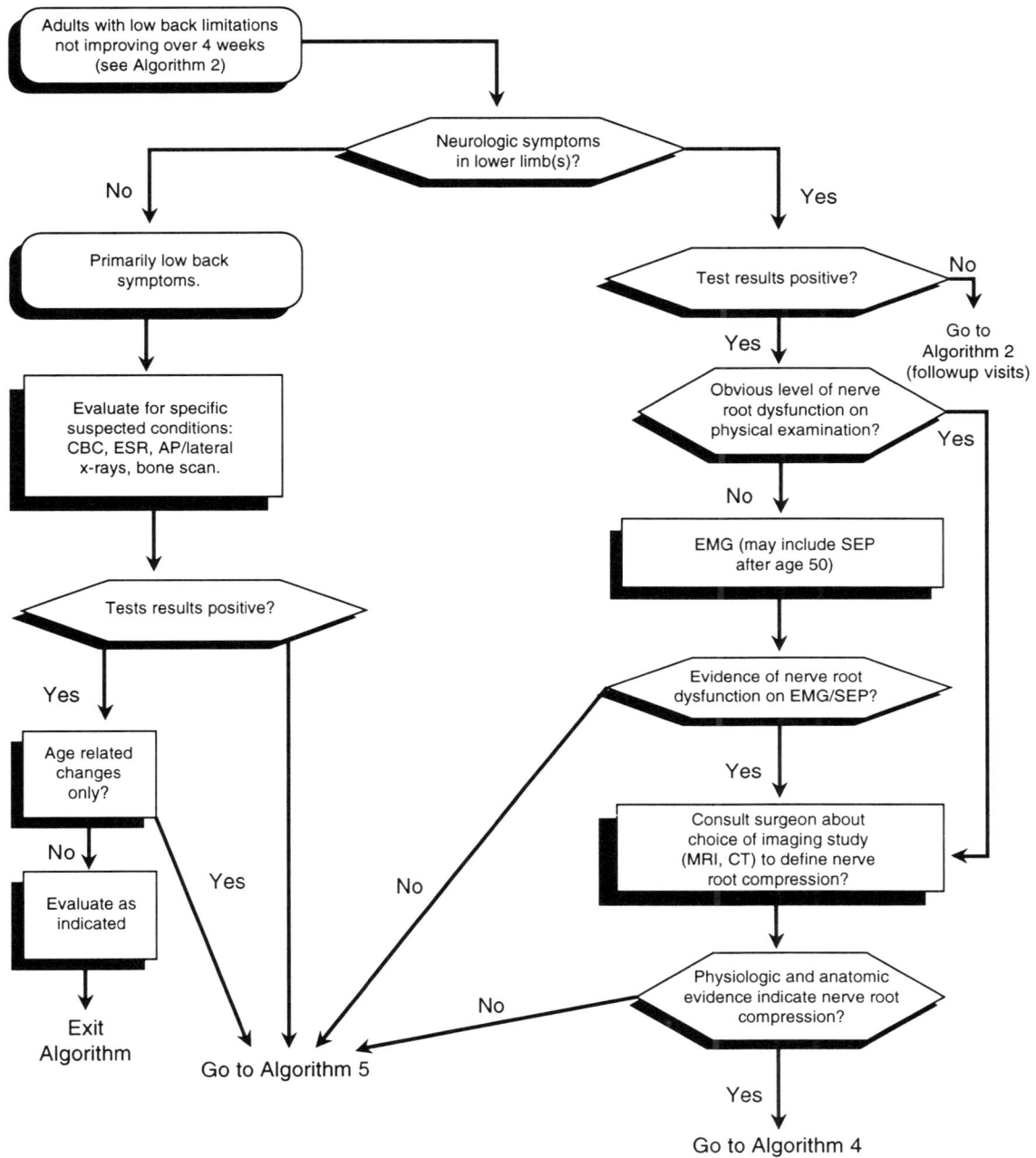

Algorithm 4   Surgical considerations for patients with persistent sciatica

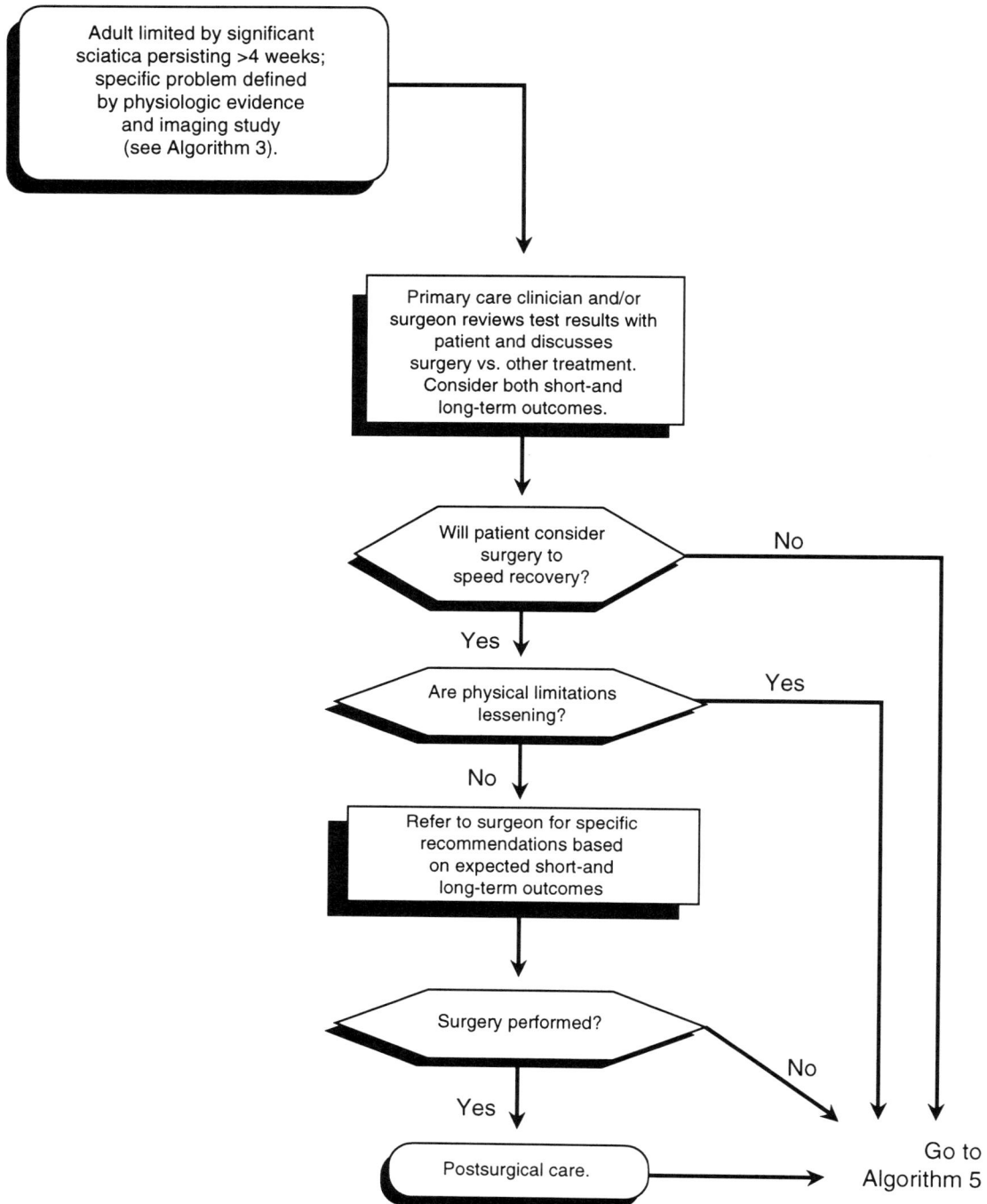

Adult limited by significant sciatica persisting >4 weeks; specific problem defined by physiologic evidence and imaging study (see Algorithm 3).

Primary care clinician and/or surgeon reviews test results with patient and discusses surgery vs. other treatment. Consider both short-and long-term outcomes.

Will patient consider surgery to speed recovery?

No

Yes

Are physical limitations lessening?

Yes

No

Refer to surgeon for specific recommendations based on expected short-and long-term outcomes

Surgery performed?

No

Yes

Postsurgical care.

Go to Algorithm 5

Table 3. Guidelines for sitting and unassisted lifting

	Severe	Moderate	Mild	None
Sitting[1]	20 min			50 min
Unassisted lifting[2]				
Men	20 lbs	20 lbs	60 lbs	80 lbs
Women	20 lbs	20 lbs	35 lbs	40 lbs

[1] Without getting up and moving around.
[2] Modification of NIOSH Lifting Guidelines, 1981, 1993. Gradually increase unassisted lifting limits to 60lbs (men) and 35lbs (women) by 3 months even with continued symptoms. Instruct patient to limit twisting, bending, reaching while lifting and to hold lifted object as close to navel as possible.

Table 4. Ability of different techniques to identify and define pathology

Technique	Indentify physiologic insult	Define anatomic defect
History	+	+
Physical examination:		
Circumference		
measurements	+	+
Reflexes	++	++
Straight leg raising (SLR)	++	+
Crossed SLR	+++	++
Motor	++	++
Sensory	++	++
Laboratory studies		
(ESR, CBC, UA)	++	0
Bone scan [1]	+++	++
EMG/SEP	+++	++
X-ray [1]	0	+
CT [1]	0	++++ [2]
MRI	0	++++ [2]
Myelo-CT [1]	0	++++ [2]
Myelography [1]	0	++++ [2]

[1] Risk of complications (radiation, infection, etc.): highest for myelo-CT, second highest for myelography, and relatively less risk for bone scan, x-ray, and CT.
[2] False-positive diagnostic findings in up to 30 percent of people without symptoms at age 30.
Note: Number of plus signs indicates relative ability to indentify or define.

Algorithm 5   Further management of acute low back problem

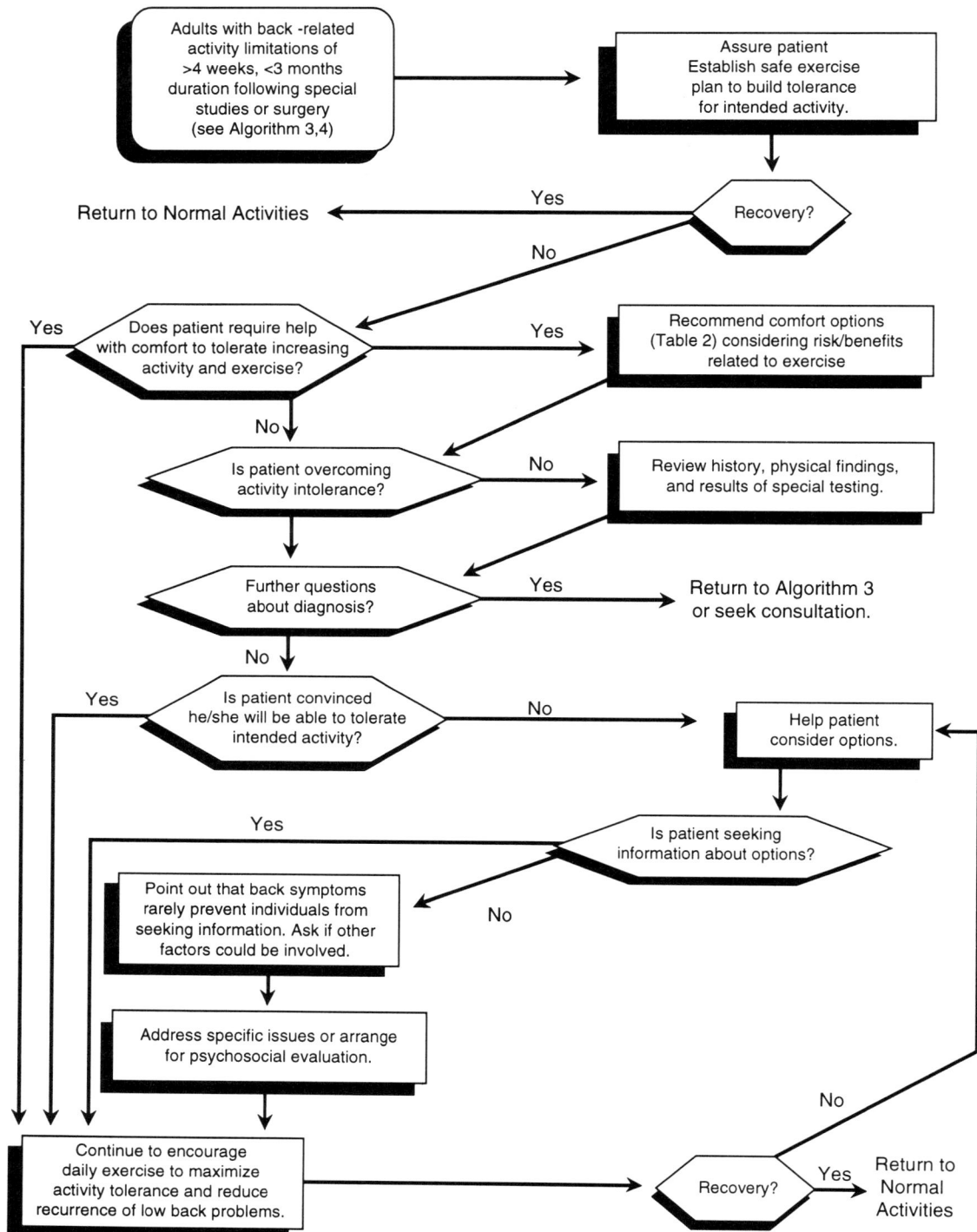

Adults with back -related
activity limitations of
>4 weeks, <3 months
duration following special
studies or surgery
(see Algorithm 3,4)

Assure patient
Establish safe exercise
plan to build tolerance
for intended activity.

Recovery?

Yes → Return to Normal Activities

No

Does patient require help
with comfort to tolerate increasing
activity and exercise?

Yes → Recommend comfort options
(Table 2) considering risk/benefits
related to exercise

No

Is patient overcoming
activity intolerance?

No → Review history, physical findings,
and results of special testing.

Further questions
about diagnosis?

Yes → Return to Algorithm 3
or seek consultation.

No

Is patient convinced
he/she will be able to tolerate
intended activity?

No → Help patient
consider options.

Is patient seeking
information about options?

Yes

No

Point out that back symptoms
rarely prevent individuals from
seeking information. Ask if other
factors could be involved.

Address specific issues or arrange
for psychosocial evaluation.

Continue to encourage
daily exercise to maximize
activity tolerance and reduce
recurrence of low back problems.

Recovery?

Yes → Return to
Normal
Activities

No

Table 5. Summary of Guideline Recommendations

The ratings in parentheses indicate the scientific evidence supporting each recommendation according to the following scale:

A = strong research-based evidence (multiple relevant and high-quality scientific studies).

B = moderate research-based evidence (one relevant, high-quality scientific study or multiple adequate scientific studies).

C = limited research-based evidence (at least one adequate scientific study in patients with low back pain).

D = panel interpretation of evidence not meeting inclusion criteria for research-based evidence.

The number of studies meeting panel review criteria is noted for each category.

	Recommend	Option	Recommend against
History and physical exam 34 studies	Basic history (B). History of cancer/ infection (B). Signs/symptoms of cauda equina syndrome (C). History of significant trauma (C). Psychosocial history (C). Straight leg raising test (B). Focused neurological exam (B).	Pain drawing and visual analog scale (D).	
Patient education 14 studies	Patient education about low back symptoms (B). Back school in occupational settings (c).	Back school in non-occupational settings (C).	
Medication 23 studies	Acetaminophen (C). NSAIDs (B).	Muscle relaxants (C). Opioids, short course (C).	Opioids used >2 wks (C). Phenylbutazone (C). Oral steroids (C). Colchicine (B). Antidepressants (C).
Physical treatment methods 42 studies	Manipulation of low back during first month of symptoms (B).	Manipulation for patients with radiculopathy (C). Manipulation for patients with symptoms >1 month (C). Self-application of heat or cold to low back. Shoe insoles (C). Corset for prevention in occupational setting (C).	Manipulation for patients with undiagnosed neurologic deficits (D). Prolonged course of manipulation (D). Traction (B). TENS (C). Biofeedback (C). Shoe lifts (D). Corset for treatment (D).
Injections 26 studies		Epidural steroid injections for radicular pain to avoid surgery (C).	Epidural injections for back pain without radiculopathy (D). Trigger point injections (C). Ligamentous injections (C). Facet joint injections (C). Needle acupuncture (D).

	Recommend	Option	Recommend against
Bed rest 4 studies		Bed rest of 2-4 days for severe radiulopathy (D).	Bed rest > 4 days (B).
Activities and exercise 20 studies	Temporary avoidance of activities that increase mechanical stress on spine (D). Gradual return to normal activities (B). Low-stress aerobic exercise (C). Conditioning exercises for trunk muscles after 2 weeks (C). Exercise quotas (C).		Back-specific exercise machines (D). Therapeutic stretching of back muscles (D).
Detection of physiologic abnormalities 14 studies	If no improvement after 1 month, consider: Bone scan (C). Needle EMG and H-reflex tests to clarify nerve root Dysfunction (C). SEP to assess spinal stenosis (C).		EMG for clinically obvious radiculopathy (D). Surface EMG and F-wave tests (C). Thermography (C).
X-rays of L-S spine 18 studies	When red flags for fracture present (C). When red flags for cancer or infection present (C).		Routine use in first month of symptoms in absence of red flags (B). Routine oblique views (B).
Imaging 18 studies	CT or MRI when cauda equina, tumor, infection, or fracture strongly suspected (C). MRI test of choice for patients with prior back surgery (D). Assure quality criteria for imaging tests (B).	Myelography or CT-myelography for preoperative planning (D).	Use of imagimg test before one month in absence red flags (B). Discography or CT-discography (C).
Surgical considerations 14 studies	Discuss surgical options with patients with persistent and severe sciatica and clinical evidence of nerve root compromise after 1 month of conservative therapy (B). Standard discectomy and microdiscectomy of similar efficacy in treatment of herinated disc (B). Chymopapain, used after ruling out allergic sensitivity, acceptable but less efficacious than discectomy to treat herniated disc (C).		Disc surgery in patients with back pain alone, no red flags, and no nerve root compression (D). Percutaneous discectomy less efficacious than chymopapain (C). Surgery for spinal stenosis within the first 3 months of symptoms (D). Stenosis surgery when justified by imaging test rather than patient's functional status (D). Spinal fusion during the first 3 months of symptoms in the absence of fracture, dislocation, complications of tumor or infection (C).
Psychosocial factors	Social, economic, and psychological factors can alter patient response to symptoms and treatment (D).		Referral for extensive evaluation/treatment prior to exploring patient expectations or psychosocial factors (D).

Treatment Guidelines:
State of New Jersey
1993

GUIDELINES FOR MANAGEMENT OF ACUTE CONDITIONS

Types of CONDITION	Levels of CARE	FREQUENCY	DURATION
Mild	Relief Therapeutic Rehabilitative Supportive	Daily visits to 3 visits per week 3 visits per week to 1 visit per week None None	1-15 days or longer 0-30 days or longer None None
Moderate	Relief Therapeutic Rehabilitative Supportive	Daily visits to 3 visits per week 3 visits per week to 1 visit per week 1 visit a week to 2 visits per month 2 visits per month to 1 visit per month	7-21 days or longer 30-60 days or longer 30-60 days or longer 0-3 months or longer
Severe	Relief Therapeutic Rehabilitative Supportive	Daily visits to 3 visits per week 3 visits per week to 1 visit per week 1 visit a week to 2 visits per month 2 visits per month to 1 visit per month	21-45 days or longer 30-90 days or longer 45-90 days or longer 3-5 months or longer

Treatment Guidelines:
State of New Jersey
1993

GUIDELINES FOR MANAGEMENT OF CHRONIC CONDITIONS

Types of CONDITION	Levels of CARE	FREQUENCY	DURATION
Mild	Relief Therapeutic Rehabilitative Supportive	None 3 visits per week to 2 visit per week 2 visits per week to 2 visits per month 2 visits per month to 1 visit per month	None 14-45 days or longer 45-90 days or longer 3-6 months or longer
Moderate	Relief Therapeutic Rehabilitative Supportive	Daily visits to 3 visits per week 3 visits per week to 2 visit per week 2 visit a week to 2 visits per month 2 visits per month to 1 visit per month	14-45 days or longer 45-90 days or longer 90-180 days or longer 6-12 months or longer
Severe	Relief Therapeutic Rehabilitative Supportive	Daily visits to 3 visits per week 3 visits per week to 2 visit per week 2 visit a week to 2 visits per month 2 visits per month to 1 visit per 3 months	30-60 days or longer 60-120 days or longer 90-180 days or longer 6-18 months or longer

Comparison Fee Facts VS. State of Hawaii
UTILIZATION GUIDELINES

Procedural Utilization Facts A.KA. Fee Facts			State of Hawaii 1000 Bishop St., Suite 601 Honolulu, Hawaii 808-537-5722	
Diagnosis	Average Treatment Time	Total Visits	Average Treatment Time	Total Visits
Acute Spinal Strain				
-mild	2-4 weeks	6-12	2-6 weeks	6-16
-moderate	8-12 weeks	20-28	8-16 weeks	20-36
-severe	12-24 weeks	28-38	12-32	28-58
Acute Spinal Sprain				
-mild	6-8 weeks	14-20	6-10 weeks	14-26
-moderate	12-14 weeks	28-38	12-32 weeks	28-50
-severe	usually requires surgery		usually requires surgery	
Chronic spinal Strain or Sprain	16-24 weeks	34-42	16-32 weeks	34-56
Torticollis				
-mild	2-4 weeks	6-12	2-6 weeks	6-16
-moderate	4-6 weeks	10-14	4-8 weeks	10-18
-severe	6-10 weeks	14-20	6-14 weeks	14-46
Cervicobrachial Syndrome	8-14 weeks	20-30	8-18 weeks	20-40
Cervicocranial Syndrome	8-14 weeks	20-30	8-16 weeks	30-36
Neurovascular Headache				
-acute	2-4 weeks	5-10	2-6 weeks	14
-chronic	10-16	22-32	10-22 weeks	22-42
-migraine	12-20	28-36	12-26 weeks	28-48
Cervicalgia	3-4 weeks	10-14	4-8 weeks	10-18
	8-12 weeks	25-35	8-16 weeks	26-46
Brachial Neuritis or Radiculitis	14-20 weeks	30-36	14-26 wweks	30-48
Cervical or Thoracic Disc Syndrome/ Displacement				
-protrusion	10-16 weeks	25-35	10-22 weeks	26-46
-herniation			16-52 weeks	36-96
-sequestered			May require surgery	
Lumbago/Lumbalgia	4-8 weeks	10-18	4-19 weeks	10-24
Sciatic Neuralgia	6-10 weeks	14-24	6-14 weeks	14-32
Lumbar Facet Syndrome	8-12 weeks	25-35	8-16 weeks	26-46
Lumbosacral or Sciatic Neuritis/Radiculitis	14-20 weeks	30-38	14-26 weeks	30-50
Spondylolisthesis				
-Grade 1	8-10 weeks	20-25	8-14 weeks	20-34
-Grade 2, 3	14-22 weeks	30-40	14-30 weeks	30-52
-Grade 4	Requires surgical intervention		Usually requires surgery	

Comparison Fee Facts VS. State of Hawaii
UTILIZATION GUIDELINES

Fee Facts   **State of Hawaii**

Diagnosis	Average Treatment Time	Total Visits	Average Treatment Time	Total Visits
Lumbar Disc Syndrome/ Displacement				
-protrusion	12-20 weeks	25-45	12-26 weeks	36-60
-herniation			20-60 weeks	36-60
-sequestered			May require surgery	
Intercostal Neuralgia				
	8-12 weeks	14-20	6-10 weeks	14-26
Intercostal Neuritis	8-12 weeks	20-28	8-16 weeks	20-36
Sacrococcygeal				
Strain/Sprain	2-6 weeks	5-14	2-8 weeks	6-18
Coccygodynia				
-acute	6-10 weeks	10-20	4-10 weeks	10-26
-chronic	12-20 weeks	28-28	12-32 weeks	22-48
Hypo or Hyper Lordosis: Cervical/Lumbar or Hyper Thoracic Kyphosis				
	4-6 weeks	4-6	4-18 weeks	4-8
Scoliosis Patients over 20 years of age				
-mild	4-6 weeks	4-6	4-8 weeks	4-8
-moderate	6-8 weeks	6-8	6-10 weeks	6-10
-severe	10-16 weeks	8-12		
Scoliosis Patients under 20 years of age				
-mild			8-16 weeks	18-32
-moderate			12-32 weeks	24-48
-severe			24-48 weeks	36-62
Degenerative Joint Disease				
-mild	4-8 weeks	4-8	4-8 weeks	4-8
-moderate	8-12 weeks	8-12	8-12 weeks	8-12
-severe	12-20 weeks	12-20	12-24 weeks	12-24
Post Laminectomy Syndrome Failed Back Surgery Syndrome				
	12-24 weeks	12-24	12-32 weeks	12-32
Ligamentous Hypermobility				
	4-8 weeks	4-8	4-10 weeks	4-10
Osteoarthritis				
	8-16 weeks	8-16	8-22 weeks	8-22

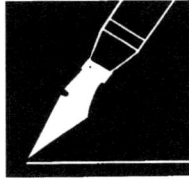

CHAPTER • ELEVEN

ANCILLARY DIAGNOSTIC PROCEDURES

OVERVIEW

All diagnostic procedures are judged based upon their ability to contribute to the differential diagnosis, prognosis, or therapeutic plan. Diagnostic tests are ordered only after a history and appropriate clinical examination are performed. They are not ordered to reassure the clinician but must contribute to the clinical picture and affect management decisions. Accuracy of a procedure is based on the ability of a procedure to determine between those who have a particular condition and those who do not (aids in differential diagnosis).

All diagnostic procedures follow patient consent and a rationale documenting the medical necessity of the test. Certain tests are dependent on patient motivation, patient cooperation, and the stage of the condition. For example, an isometric muscle testing evaluation should not be done in an acute condition due to the pain, restriction of motion, and the potential for causing further injury.

The information gained from a test may change the diagnosis or indicate a need for a change in therapy. The efficacy of a test is the ability of the test to reduce diagnostic uncertainty. The test must contribute to the differential diagnosis, therapeutic plan, and prognosis. Also, the history and examination may not indicate the need for a diagnostic procedure, but the diagnostic imaging is used to assess for contraindications to certain therapeutic approaches. All procedures should be chosen judiciously based on accepted professional standards. The benefit of the test must outweigh any associated risks involved with the procedure and the report of findings must be given in a timely manner.

Terminology for diagnostic imaging and instrumentation includes:

1. *Validity:* The property of information derived from a test or measurement that assures it represents the desired function.

2. *Accuracy:* The property of a measurement which determines how closely the result will approximate the truth.

3. *Discriminability:* The property of information derived from a test or a measurement allows the practitioner to discern between groups of subjects; for example, healthy from unhealthy.

4. *Reliability:* The ability to obtain the same measurement of a stable function or structure upon repeated tests. Reliability depends both on accuracy and precision which may be separately evaluated and adjusted for calibration.

5. *Sensitivity:* The ability to correctly identify positive test results among subjects who truly have a specific disorder. The likelihood of a positive test result in a person with a disorder.

6. *Specificity:* The ability to correctly identify negative test results among subjects who truly do not have a specific disorder. The likelihood of a negative test result in a patient without a disorder.

CLINICALLY NECESSARY CRITERIA (Mercy):

Services and supplies which are determined to be:

1. Appropriate and necessary for the symptom, diagnosis/clinical impression, or care/treatment of the patient condition;

2. Provided for the diagnosis/clinical impression, or to direct care and treatment of the health care condition;

3. According to standards of good primary health care practice within the organized professional community;

4. Not primarily for the convenience of the patient, or one or more of the patient's providers; and

5. The most appropriate supply or level of service.

ADDITIONAL CRITERIA

6. Documented in the patient's records in a reasonable manner, including the relationship of the diagnosis to the service.

7. For Worker's Compensation and automobile insurance coverage, the service must be useful and medically appropriate to restore and rehabilitate a patient to his preinjury state or to achieve a reasonable, maximum benefit.

8. Be evaluated for efficacy on a regular basis and modified in a meaningful fashion to reflect patient response or the lack thereof.

REVIEWING DIAGNOSTIC IMAGING AND INSTRUMENTATION

A negative test does not mean that the test was not indicated by the clinical findings. If there is question in the reviewer's mind about the medical necessity of a test, the reviewer should respect the judgment of the ordering clinician. Some of the following questions may assist you in determining whether a procedure is medically necessary:

1. Did the procedure aid in the determination of a differential diagnosis, prognosis, or contribute to the therapeutic plan?

2. What was the rationale for ordering the test in question?

3. Did the test follow an appropriate history and clinical examination?

4. Should have the test been delayed in favor of seeking a second opinion evaluation?

5. Did the benefit of the test outweigh the risks associated with the test?

6. Is the procedure reasonable according to the accepted standards of care?

PLAIN FILM X-RAY (SECTIONAL STUDIES)

Plain film x-rays are commonly used in chiropractic practice. Greater than 50% of all practicing chiropractors have their own in-office x-ray units. X-rays are used to rule out fracture, dislocation, or gross osseous pathology. An appropriate history and clinical examination are used to determine the appropriate area(s) to x-ray and the views to be taken. The benefit of the test must out weigh the risk. This procedure provides a low cost means of evaluating musculoskeletal injuries and is usually the first imaging test performed. X-rays should not be taken just to "reassure" the doctor, but follow a rationale for performing the study. Only the areas of clinical interest should be x-rayed.

A minimum x-ray series includes two views at right angles of each other. Extra views can be added as indicated clinically. Single views may be exposed within six weeks after a complete series has been taken. Repeat studies should be used only when indicated clinically. Repeat x-rays may be used to assess for an advancing underlying pathology, monitoring of a fracture, monitoring a scoliosis, or when there is significant reinjury or exacerbation. Repeat x-rays must be medically necessary. X-rays should not be routinely exposed on patients. Factors such as the patient's age, pregnancy, and radiation therapy should be assessed before x-rays are taken. X-rays also may be used to assess for clinically silent conditions that may serve as contraindications to certain forms of therapy. The clinical findings may not warrant x-ray exposure, but the choice of technique requires the clinician to assess for clinically silent conditions.

Stress x-rays can be used in evaluating for abnormal joint motion and spinal instability. The AMA Guides the the Evaluation of Permanent Impairment recommends using stress films in assessing impairments. There is, however, some question of the influence of stress films on the clinical management of mechanical back syndromes. Some authors suggest using stress films and a templating system to document soft tissue injuries following traumatic injuries such as whiplash.

PLAIN FILM X-RAY (FULL SPINE)

Full spine x-rays are used in Chiropractic to evaluate and monitor a scoliosis and for biomechanical assessment. Full spine x-rays are not appropriate for assessing a patient post-trauma since sectional studies are the standard for trauma assessment. Full spine x-ray usage is limited to biomechanical assessments and scoliosis monitoring. Certain techniques in chiropractic, such as Gonstead, advocate the use of full spine x-rays for analytical purposes.

This study may be a common procedure involved in utilization review. Third party payers ask if they should have to pay for the entire spine when a specific injury was related to only one area of the spine. The third party payer is responsible for only the area of the spine relating to the specific injury.

VIDEOFLUOROSCOPY

This procedure is a functional joint study to evaluate for biomechanical abnormality. This procedure is not new and requires an examiner who is skilled to interpret the findings.

This test may be useful in cases of ligamentous instability, spinal stenosis, postoperative evaluation, flexion/extension injuries, presumed radicular compression, and when hypermobility cannot be detected by plain film x-rays. This test should not be routinely used.

The examiner must ask whether the risk of this test outweighs the exposure and if the outcome of this study will affect the treatment or case management. There must also be consideration to reliable tests that are less hazardous.

DIAGNOSTIC ULTRASOUND/SPINAL SONOGRAM

This procedure has been the center of much controversy in recent years. The use of diagnostic ultrasound has been established for many years in evaluating soft tissues of the abdomen, musculoskeletal structures including rotator cuff tears and other superficial structures, and in pediatrics. The use of diagnostic ultrasound in the adult spine is still considered investigational and seems to be primarily limited to the chiropractic profession.

There is very little, if any, sound evidence in the scientific literature regarding the use of diagnostic ultrasound in evaluating adult spinal structures. Operator skill and reproducible technique are important to the outcome of the test. The type of equipment used is also very important. Who reads the scans? A highly qualified doctor is needed to read the scans. This training requires intensive training in proper anatomy as well as having read hundreds of ultrasound scans. Diagnostic ultrasound should not be used to replace a thorough clinical examination to diagnose sprain/strain injuries. The use of the diagnostic ultrasound must have an effect on the clinical management.

ACA position on Diagnostic Ultrasound: " Diagnostic ultrasound has been shown to be a useful modality for evaluating certain musculoskeletal complaints. The quality of US images is extremely dependent on operator skill. The resolution abilities of the equipment may have an impact on diagnostic yield and accuracy. Consequently, the importance of training to establish technologic as well as interpretative competency cannot be understated. The application of diagnostic US in the adult spine in the areas such as disc herniation, spinal stenosis, and nerve root pathology is inadequately studied and its routine application for these purposes cannot be supported by the evidence at this time."

The American College of Radiology: "The use of diagnostic spinal ultrasound in the evaluation of pain or radiculopathy syndromes (facet joints and capsules, nerve and fascial edema, and other subtle paraspinal abnormalities) currently has no proven clinical utility as a screening, diagnostic, or adjunctive screening tool."

MAGNETIC RESONANCE IMAGING/ MRI

The MRI is used to evaluate soft tissue structures and bone in one image. This study shows nerve roots, discs, bone, and other soft tissue structures. This test should not be used for routine screening due to the cost. Due to the high cost of the MRI, plain film x-rays and other lower cost analytical measures are typically performed first. The utilization of this procedure must meet the medically necessary criteria.

COMPUTERIZED TOMOGRAPHY/CT SCAN

This test can be equally as sensitive when evaluating spinal structures but this procedure is more invasive than MRI. CT is used to visualize planes not visible on plain film radiography. Indications for CT include: evaluating the cervicothoracic junction, further evaluation of a fracture or dislocation seen on plain film x-rays, and the presence of neurologic symptoms whose cause cannot be determined by plain film x-ray. CT follows plain film x-rays and is very reliable for assessing bone and disc pathology. CT should not be used as a routine screening procedure.

ELECTRODIAGNOSTIC TESTING

Select neuromuscular dysfunction is detected by these studies. Electrodiagnostic studies are used to evaluate both the central and peripheral nervous systems. The stage and severity of the condition must be considered when determining whether these studies will affect the treatment management or contribute to a differential diagnosis in a given case. Surface or needle electrodes can be used, but needle electrodes help decrease variables and increase reliability.

1. *Nerve Conduction Studies:* This test evaluates for nerve trunk integrity and can be done by using either a needle or surface electrode. It is reliable with both the sensitivity and specificity being well studied. Sensory or motor nerves can be measured for dysfunction. Motor nerves can be evaluated for dysfunction from mechanical or pathological causes. Clinical examination is used to establish the need for this test. This test may be delayed in favor of pursuing a neurological consultation. The NCV is typically used in conjunction with the EMG. This procedure is used for some of the following conditions in chiropractic: carpal tunnel syndrome, ulnar neuropathies, peroneal neuropathies, brachial plexus lesions, and radiculopathy (cervical or lumbar).

2. *Electromyelography (Needle electrode):* This test measures the electrical activity of skeletal muscle. Denervation may take up to six weeks to become evident in distal muscles due to slow progression of axonal degeneration. For this reason, the EMG test is usually delayed following acute trauma. Sensory peripheral lesions may not be detected with the EMG. This test is established by clinical examination. The EMG is used to confirm and determine the precise location of radicular findings evident on the clinical examination. This test is typically used to differentiate nerve root lesions from plexopathies, determine precise level of radicular involvement, and evaluating myopathies.

3. *Somatosensory Evoked Potentials/SSEP:* This test evaluates the sensory part of the nervous system. It will follow the appropriate clinical examination. This test is becoming more important in the evaluation of radiculopathy since

many radicuolpathies are purely sensory in nature. It will also be used for detection of dysfunction not previously found by other electrodiagnostic studies. This test is used for the detection of sensory nerve disorders, myelopathy, thoracic outlet syndrome, and multiple sclerosis.

SURFACE ELECTROMYELOGRAPHY/SEMG

This test measures asymmetry of spinal muscles. This procedure is considered by most authors an investigational procedure. The SEMG is subject to high variables and the impact on treatment management and differential diagnosis has not yet been established. This procedure has been advocated by some to be used for "outcome assessment," but the medical necessity as a diagnostic procedure has not been established.

A baseline evaluation is usually followed by one or more repeat studies. Typically, clinicians will never refer to this test in their documentation or indicate how this test has influenced treatment management of contributed to a differential diagnosis.

MUSCLE TESTING

Measurement of strength can be done by low-cost hand-held dynamometers to high cost sophisticated equipment. Hand-held units are more variable than certain other types of testing devices. Acute conditions are contraindications to testing because of muscle spasm, pain, and the risk of causing further inflammation. A difference of at least 20% may be needed when evaluating patient performance. There are three types of testing: isometric, isokinetic, and isoinertial.

1. *Isometric testing:* Depends on inertial effects at the onset of the test, patient fatigue, posture, and motivation. Bilateral differences greater than 15-20% indicate abnormality.

2. *Isokinetic testing:* The primary measurement is a torque generated which is only valid during the controlled part of motion.

3. *Isoinertial testing:* Can be made capable of motoring position, velocity, and torque simultaneously.

   Contraindications to testing include: spinal instability, severe osteoporosis, inflammatory spondyloarthropathy, unstable spondylolisthesis, progressive neurological deficits, heart disease, and spinal tumors.

These tests may be used for preparedness to return to work, setting treatment goals, or to judge the therapeutic benefit of a rehabilitation program. Muscle testing is typically done prior to initiating a strength rehabilitation program, six weeks after the initiation of the program, and at any time when the information gathered will affect a change in therapeutic protocols.

THERMOGRAPHY

This procedure is used to detect slight changes in skin temperature. These studies follow strict protocols and guidelines to minimize variables and guidelines. These examinations are also time-consuming and require a highly trained professional to administer and interpret the test. The primary application is to demonstrate sensory nerve involvement. This is the procedure of choice for the evaluation of Reflex Sympathetic Dystrophy. The medical necessity of this test is judged by its ability to affect treatment management and aid in differential diagnosis.

THERMOCOUPLE DEVICE

These are widely used in the chiropractic profession. They are hand-held devices designed to detect temperature variations of local paraspinal areas, and are highly variable. The use of these devices is included in the charges for the adjustment or office visit. These devices are not medically necessary as a separate and distinct diagnostic procedure.

PRESSURE ALGOMETRY

This device has gained some popularity in recent years. This measures pain threshold applied to myofascial structures. Pressure is applied until the patient perceives pain. The pressure required to produce pain is recorded for several different sites.

MEASUREMENT OF MOVEMENT/RANGE OF MOTION/ GONIOMETER/INCLINOMETRY

These procedures are widely used in health care. Range of motion is one of the components of an examination. Goniometers are accurate to a range of 10-15 degrees. Inclinometers are more accurate and range from 3-5 degrees. These procedures are bundled in the fee for the examination and are not typically billed for separately. The use of these procedures being done as part on an impairment rating requested by an insurance carrier or attorney would justify separate billing.

ROENTGENOGRAPHIC FINDINGS OF THE CERVICAL SPINE IN "ASYMPTOMATIC PEOPLE," *SPINE*, VOL. 11, #6, 1986

By the age of 60-65, 95% of men and 70% of women had at least one degenerative change on roentgenograms. Cervical spondylosis is a common x-ray finding in asymptomatic people. Structural changes evident on x-ray do not necessarily cause symptoms.

ABNORMAL MAGNETIC RESONANCE SCANS OF THE LUMBAR SPINE IN "ASYMPTOMATIC SUBJECTS," *J. OF BONE AND JOINT SURGERY*, 1990

Abnormalities on MRI must be strictly correlated with age and any clinical signs and symptoms before operative treatment is contemplated. Substantial percentages of individuals who never had low back pain or sciatica but had abnormal Myelograms (24%), CT (36%), or Discograms (37%) have been reported. In the present study, 30% of an asymptomatic population had a major abnormality on a MRI of the lumbar spine.

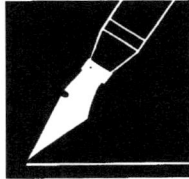

CHAPTER • TWELVE

SOFT TISSUE INJURY AND REPAIR

This chapter provides the basic knowledge each doctor needs when understanding the healing process of soft tissues. This will better allow the clinician to explain the healing process to his/her patients, insurance carriers, and attorneys. An understanding of the healing process also allows for selection of appropriate treatment and modalities. I would suggest acquiring a few of the reference articles found at the end of this text for a complete study on the healing process. Knowledge of the stages of healing and soft tissue repair is essential for the selection of the appropriate adjunctive modalities. There are three phases to soft tissue healing:

PHASE 1/ACUTE OR INFLAMMATORY PHASE

This is the first step in the healing of injured tissues and will last up to 72 hours. The cells involved during this time are brought to the injured area by the circulatory system. Histamine is released which results in vasodilation and the classic signs of the inflammatory response (redness, swelling, heat, and pain). Prostaglandins also contribute to long term vasodilation. A fibrin plug is formed to prevent against blood loss. Healing will not begin without inflammation but excess inflammation will lead to excess scar formation. Phagocytosis is the process that gets rid of the infection and decontaminates the wound.

White blood cells such as polymorphonuclear leukocytes and macrophages are involved in this phase of healing. The macrophages ingest the bacteria and influence the number of repair cells that will be involved. Anti-inflammatory steroids can inhibit the white blood cells during this time.

New blood vessels are needed to supply oxygen and nutrients to the healing tissues. The production of new blood vessels is called neovascularization. Immobilization is limited to 3-4 days but is used to prevent microhemmorrhage. Active exercise should be avoided during this time. Heat during this phase would also cause increased bleeding and an increased inflammatory response. The treatment of choice would be PRICE (protection, rest, ice, compression, and elevation).

Using ice in the inflammatory phase has several advantages. Ice can be effective for localized pain control as well as reducing disability. Applying cryotherapy within the first 24 hours is very effective in decreasing the overall treatment time of an injury. Conversely, not using cryotherapy soon enough may lengthen the treatment time. Healing is also influenced by any pre-injury medications and disease processes. The classic signs of an acute inflammatory response are usually not present in a chronic overuse condition or repetitive microtrauma, even though the inflammation is proceeding at the microscopic level.

PHASE 2/FIBROPLASTIC OR REPAIR PHASE

This will last from 48 hours to 6 weeks. The cell primarily responsible for scar formation is called the fibroblast. Once the wound has been cleaned, collagen production starts and may last up to six weeks depending on the severity of the injury. This is the body's attempt to regenerate the damaged tissue. If the wound has not been cleaned, the synthesis of collagen does not take place. Ascorbic acid, zinc, iron, copper, and oxygen are all needed to help in the formation of collagen.

Cross-links form to impart strength to the wound but the collagen is not completely organized. Complications can cause a recurrence of the inflammation and should be avoided. Passive exercises are started during this phase of healing. Early passive exercises help maintain neurologic pathways. Some authors suggest that maximum recovery will not take place if appropriate exercises are between weeks 3 and 14 are not done.

PHASE 3/REMODELING PHASE

This lasts from 3 weeks to 12 months or more depending on the extent of the injury. The tensile strength of the collagen is dependent on the forces placed on it during this time. Controlled forces are used to influence scar formation and increase its functional capabilities. Rehabilitative exercises are used to duplicate stresses to which the tissues will be exposed to. Scar tissue is less resilient, less elastic, and less resistant to tensile forces than "normal" tissue.

Immobilization should be avoided during this time. Early mobilization minimizes muscle wasting and strength loss, minimizes risk for re-injury, minimizes adhesions that may prevent movement, helps maintain joint proprioception, and assists in the nutrition of soft tissues. Pain during the rehabilitative process should not be ignored or masked by using ice or medications. Pain during rehabilitative exercise may indicate that further damage is being done.

ETIOLOGY OF SOFT TISSUE INJURIES (KELLET)

1. Direct injuries are usually due to blunt trauma and occur more frequently in body contact sports, e.g., muscle contusion, eye injuries, lacerations, and cerebral concussions.

2. Indirect injuries which may be further subdivided into:

    a. *Acute*—Occurs with sudden overloading of musculo-tendinous units, as might occur in sprinting or kicking resulting, e.g., in "torn muscles."

    b. *Chronic or overuse*—Due to repeated overload and/or frictional resistance which occurs in endurance training or other highly repetitive action, e.g., tendinitis.

    c. *Acute on chronic*—Due to a sudden rupture of a persistent lesion, e.g., rupture of a chronic achilles tendinitis.

SEVERITY (KELLET)

1. *Grade 1 (first degree):* Mild pain at the time of the injury or within 24 hours of injury, especially when stress is applied to the injury; local tenderness may or may not be present.

2. *Grade2 (second degree):* The person notices pain during activity and usually has to stop; pain and local tenderness are moderate to severe when the injury is stressed.

3. *Grade 3 (third degree):* Complete or near complete rupture or avulsion of at least a portion of a ligament or tendon with severe pain or loss of function; a palpable defect may be present; stressing a ruptured ligament may, paradoxically, be painless due to the loss of continuity of the tissue.

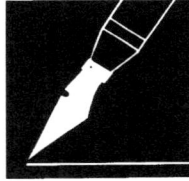

CHAPTER • THIRTEEN

ADJUNCTIVE PROCEDURES

An understanding of the healing process (Chapter 12) is essential prior to determining adjunctive modalities. A clinician must understand the healing process that is taking place before procedures can be chosen. The modalities are chosen with respect to the stage of healing and the desired physiologic response. These procedures should not be utilized until a complete history and examination is performed. Specific goals should be determined before the use of any modality.

For an in-depth study of the current guidelines in the Chiropractic profession, I would recommend the text books by the Chiropractic Rehabilitation Association and the recently published ACA Guidelines.

CLASSIFICATIONS OF MODALITIES:

We will cover some of the more frequently used modalities and their classifications. The most appropriate use of these will be determined by the phase of the healing process, clinical findings, doctor preference, and the patients response or lack of response to the treatment rendered. The classes include:

Cryotherapy: Ice packs, ice massage.

Superficial Heat: Infared, hot packs.

Deep Heat: Short wave diathermy, microwave diathermy, and ultrasound.

Electrical Muscle Stimulators: Motor and sensory stimulation, trigger point.

Traction: Flexion-distraction, intermittent, intersegmental, and continuous.

Soft Tissue: Trigger point therapy, massage, and myofascial release.

Rehabilitative Exercises: Passive, active, and work hardening.

GENERAL PRINCIPLES

The number of modalities utilized should decrease to correspond with patient progress. The selection of appropriate adjunctive modalities should be based upon the desired physiological response with consideration to the phase of healing the patient is currently in. Therapies producing the same effect should not be used at the same time unless there is appropriate documentation for the rationale of treatment. In other words, the clinician should explain why he/she is using two therapies that produce the same or similar results. Assessment for contra-indications should be made prior to the utilization of any modalities and quanti-tative assessment.

In the case of an acute moderate to severe injury, up to three adjunctive modalities in addition to spinal adjustments in the initial phase of treatment may be clinically necessary to achieve the desired response. These may include, but should not be limited to: cryotherapy, immobilization, pulsed ultrasound, bracing, interferential, high volt galvanic, microcurrent and massage. Heat is contraindicated in the acute phase of soft tissue injury under most circumstances. Excess heat may increase inflammation and scar tissue formation.

As the patient responds to treatment, the use of adjunctive modalities decreases. One to two adjunctive modalities in the middle stages of healing may be utilized. The Ohio State Chiropractic Guidelines advocate the use of no more than two modalities per visit in addition to spinal adjustments. These may include, but are not limited to: soft tissue technique, intersegmental traction, deep heat, superficial heat, interferential, and TENS.

Early controlled passive exercises should be introduced to minimize muscle wasting and facilitate maintenance of normal neurological pathways. These may include passive, passive-assistive, and passive-resistive. These would be limited to a pain free range of motion.

As the patient progresses and moves into the remodeling phase, the treatment emphasis switches from passive treatment to active treatment. One adjunctive modality in addition to spinal adjustments would be reasonable. These would include, but not be limited to: soft tissue technique and muscle stimulation such as Russian stimulation. Active rehabilitation would be initiated in the final stage of healing. An in-office rehabilitation session may last from 15 minutes to more than one hour and may be at the frequency of 3-5 times per week to achieve the desired results. This would also be switched to home-based self-treatment once pre-injury levels are reached.

RECORD KEEPING

Documentation for adjunctive modalities should include the date of service, the area of treatment, the setting, and treatment time. Any adverse or undesired reactions should also be noted in the patient's file. The initials of the person(s) administering the treatment are included as well.

Specific goals should be stated prior to a home-based or in-office rehabilitation program. These goals may include restoring muscle strength, speed, and endurance. Rehabilitation may also encompass flexibility, proprioception, and coordination. Quantitative assessments are routinely used in the rehabilitation process. Repeat testings should be compared to prior testings and these comparisons should be documented in the patient's records. (Muscle testing is covered in Chapter 11)

CONTRAINDICATIONS TO ADJUNCTIVE MODALITIES

The following tables are designed to offer a general idea of contraindications to certain adjunctive modalities. These are not entirely complete. For a complete listing of all contraindications to specific adjunctive modalities, I would suggest consulting a text book on physiologic therapeutics.

CONTRAINDICATIONS TO LOCAL HEAT

1. Fractures
2. Malignant tumors
3. Over gonads or gravid uterus
4. Acute inflammatory process
5. Extensive vascular disorders

CONTRAINDICATIONS TO COLD

1. Raynaud's phenomenon
2. When arthritic stiffness may be aggravated by cold
3. Do not apply when the patient is cold
4. Advanced age
5. Infancy

CONTRAINDICATIONS TO ULTRASOUND

1. Malignancy
2. Gonads or pregnant uterus
3. The eye
4. Growing epiphysis
5. Metal implants
6. Healing fracture
7. Vascular emboli or hemorrhage

GENERAL CONTRAINDICATIONS OF ELECTRICAL CURRENTS

1. Never through the heart, eyes, or brain
2. Over menstruating or the gravid uterus
3. Over bony prominences
4. Malignant tumors
5. Pacemaker
6. Fracture or dislocation
7. Abcess, inflammation, or hemophilia

CONTRAINDICATIONS TO MASSAGE AND OTHER SOFT TISSUE TECHNIQUES

1. Too much pain produced

2. Phlebitis, thrombitis or other vascular disease.

3. Infectious bone or joint disease

4. Acute cuts or abrasions

5. The patient dislikes the procedure

SELECTED MODALITIES

1. *Cryotherapy:* This is the procedure of choice in the acute phase of soft tissue healing. The usage of this modality is not limited to the acute phase only. The use of cold can be used in the acute, subacute, and, sometimes, the chronic phase. Some patients just do not respond to hot packs but do respond to cold or a contrast of hot and cold. The use of cold decreases pain, decreases edema, and reduces spasticity. Treatment time with commercial cold packs is 10-20 minutes and treatment time for an ice massage should not exceed 10 minutes.

2. *Hot pack:* This is considered a superficial heat. The treatment time ranges from 10-20 minutes. Some guidelines and authors suggest that this should not be billed for after one month due to the reduction of therapeutic benefit. Also, if this procedure is used for five minutes prior to an adjustment it should not be billed separately because this does not constitute a therapeutic dose.

3. *Ultrasound:* This procedure is considered a high frequency modality that can be set on continuous which is heat producing or pulsed which is non heat producing. Continuous ultrasound is contraindicated in acute injuries but pulsed ultrasound can be used in either acute or chronic conditions. The typical treatment time is 5-8 minutes. This is one of the most widely used modalities. Pulsed ultrasound produces micromassage of the tissue and continuous ultrasound produces vasodilation.

4. *Electrical Muscle Stimulatiuon (EMS):* This modality consists of different wave forms (pulsed, tetanizing, surged). The average treatment time is 5-20 minutes depending on the desired effect. This modality is used to exercise or reeducate muscles, decrease pain and edema, tone muscle tissue, and fatigue spasm.

5. *Interferential:* This is a commonly used modality for pain control. The treatment time is typically 15 minutes and tolerated better than most electrical modalities. It is commonly used when analgesia or pain control is the desired result.

6. *High Volt Galvanic:* This modality is used for muscle stimulation and is more deeply penetrating than other modalities. The average treatment time is 10-20 minutes. The uses include pain control, decreased edema, and increased muscle strength.

7. *Massage and Soft Tissue Procedures:* These may vary somewhat depending on the technique used. Treatment time can vary from 5 minutes to a half hour depending on the technique. They help reduce edema, increase range of motion, reduce scar tissue formation, decrease pain, and allow for relaxation.

8. *Intersegmental Traction:* This procedure is designed to limit adhesions by separation of the spinal joints and soft tissue attachments. The modality induces motion in the spine and usually lasts from 10-20 minutes.

9. *Orthopedic Supplies:* Under certain circumstances, the treating doctor may prescribe an orthopedic support for his/her patient. Cervical collars and cervical pillows are commonly used following whiplash injuries. A lumbar support cushion or heel lifts may be appropriate for certain low back disorders. These procedures may be used to help support, immobilize, or rehabilitate an injured area.

OHIO GUIDELINES

These guidelines were published in 1996 by the Ohio State Chiropractic Association and cover generally accepted treatment procedures for chiropractic. These guidelines were derived from the Oklahoma Workers' Compensation Guidelines, Mercy Guidelines, Rand Corporation Guidelines, and the Canadian Guidelines. Each procedure is given a optimum duration to produce its desired effects. These guidelines also recommend a switch from passive to active care as the condition is improving. A key point to these guidelines is that the patient should be reevaluated every 2-4 weeks. The guidelines also state that up to 2 modalities per injured area in addition to manipulation or an office visit is considered appropriate. This guideline states that more than 2 modalities per area per day is a red flag.

Thermal Treatment (superficial and deep heat including ultrasound, cold)

* *Treatment Frequency:* 3-5 times per week, decreasing to 2 times per week after one month

* *Optimum Duration:* 2-3 months in conjunction with other therapies

Traction

* *Optimum Duration:* 1-2 months; may continue this modality as needed (unsupervised) if this modality facilitates objective functional gains

TENS

* *Optimum Frequency:* 2 times a week for three weeks for supervised use.

* *Optimum Duration:* 1-2 months

Therapeutic Exercise

* *Time to Produce Effect:* 2-6 weeks

* *Treatment Frequency:* 2-5 times per week supervised for the first 3-4 weeks, decreasing to 2-4 times per week, thereafter for 4-8 weeks

* *Optimum Duration:* 4-8 weeks

* *Maximum Duration:* 3-4 months, exclusive of intervening medical complications

NORTH AMERICAN SPINE SOCIETY GUIDELINES

These guidelines were developed in 1993 and include common therapeutic procedures used in the treatment of lumbosacral disorders. The natural history of most lumbar spine pain syndromes is 90-120 days (3-4 months) following the initial onset of pain.

Thermal treatment

- *Treatment Frequency:* 3 times per week decreasing to 2 times per week after 1 month.
- *Maximum Duration:* 2-3 months

Traction

- *Treatment Frequency:* 2-3 times per week
- *Maximum Treatment Duration:* 1 month

Restriction of Activity

- *Treatment Frequency:* continuous
- *Optimum Treatment:* 3 days
- *Maximum Treatment Duration:* 7 days

Exercise therapy

- *Minimum time for treatment response:* 4-6 weeks
- *Treatment Frequency:* 2-6 times per week of supervised exercise for the first four weeks, decreasing to 2-4 times per week thereafter.
- *Optimum Treatment Duration:* 3-4 months
- *Maximum Treatment Duration:* 4-6 months

OKLAHOMA WORKERS' COMPENSATION LOW BACK PAIN GUIDELINES

These guidelines were developed in 1995 and included the Mercy Guidelines, AHCPR Guidelines, and North American Spine Society Guidelines. These guidelines also stress the importance of reevaluating the patient every two to four weeks to make sure that the treatment is producing positive results.

MODALITY GUIDELINES

These guidelines indicate that up to two adjunctive modalities may be performed in addition to a spinal adjustment as long as the physiologic effects do not significantly overlap. Reassessment should show significant improvement and ongoing care must be documented by continued improvement. There must also be a switch to active care.

ACTIVE INTERVENTIONS

- As the patient progresses active care is emphasized over passive modalities.
- Patient education, exercises, lifestyle modifications, and other active measures must be included if treatment extends beyond 18 visits.

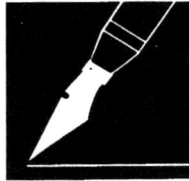

CHAPTER • FOURTEEN

MANIPULATION UNDER ANESTHESIA (MUA)

A. OVERVIEW

Manipulation Under Anesthesia has been used successfully for many years in treating acute and chronic musculoskeletal conditions. The purpose of the anesthesia is to obliterate the patient's response to pain and spasm that may limit other forms of conservative care from being successful. MUA is designed to stretch or tear the periarticular adhesions that form around the articular facets of the spine which are usually caused by time, trauma to the spine, or by herniated or bulged discs. These periarticular adhesions are what tend to lock the spine in a state of fixation, preventing normal movement and causing pain. The paraspinal muscles cause a splinting or guarding at the adhesion site which makes the traditional chiropractic manipulation less effective. The benefits of this procedure include return of normal spinal movement, the normal structural integrity of the spine is reestablished, and elimination of symptomatic pain, and an increased range of motion.

B. INDICATIONS FOR PERFORMING MANIPULATION UNDER ANESTHESIA

Indications for MUA include failure to respond to conservative chiropractic care in the office setting after a minimum of two to six weeks of continuous conservative care; chronic or recurrent pain; pain so severe that narcotic analgesics are of little value; chronic myositis; chronic fibrositis; nerve entrapment; disc pathology-herniations less than 3mm in lumbar spine documented by CT, MRI, or myelography; traumatically reduced restriction of range of motion; lumbarization or sacralization associated with acute/chronic pain; traumatic torticollis; failed spinal surgery; and headaches of nonorganic origin.

C. CONTRAINDICATIONS FOR MUA:

Contraindications of MUA include infectious bone disease; acute fractures; acute inflammatory arthiritis (gout or rheumatoid); TB of bone, gonorrheal spinal arthritis; osteoporosis; "direct" manipulation of old compression fractures; uncontrolled diabetic neuropathy; syphilitic articular or periarticular lesions; evidence of cord or caudal compression by tumor or disc herniation over 3mm in the cervical spine or 5mm in the lumbar spine; widespread staph. or strep infection; respiratory infections; metastatic bone infections; any form of malignancy or metastasis; prior history of stroke; discitis; osteogenesis imperfecta; vertebral artery syndrome; abdominal aortic syndrome; clotting disorders; and pregnancy.

D. PRE-MUA REQUIREMENTS

1. *Chiropractic:* History and physical; 2-6 weeks of care; X-rays, CT, or MRI; Other diagnostic testing

2. *Neurology/Orthopedic:* Evaluation and/or clearance for MUA; EMG/NCV, SSEP

3. *Medical:* History and physical; CBC; Possible EKG and/or chest x-ray

4. *Anesthesiology:* Anesthesia clearance

E. MUA PROCEDURE

1. Daily admission through the hospitals short stay under the control and orders of an anesthesiologist.

2. Daily pain drawings and one Oswestry disability and/or neck disability index form on the first day of admission.

3. Administration of Propofol via IV as the sedative/hypnotic.

4. Manipulation provided by a licensed chiropractor certified in MUA and a second chiropractor to serve as the first assistant. Procedure to include passive ROM stretching and manipulation to the appropriate area.

5. Recovery in the recovery room.

6. Patient released when stabilized.

7. Follow-up care in office for 7-10 days. Treatment to include hot moist packs, passive ROM stretching, interferential current and cryotherapy. After the tenth day include manipulation into the protocol (3 times weekly for 2 weeks). Then rehab 3- 4 times weekly and manipulation 1 time weekly for four weeks (Rehab. to include isometric, isotonic, and theraband). The follow-up treatment is critical to the success of the MUA.

F. NATIONAL ACADEMY OF MANIPULATION UNDER ANESTHESIA PHYSICIANS PROTOCOLS AND STANDARDS
Oct. 26 and 27, 1996 Atlanta, Georgia

1. **Clinical Justification**

   Clinical justification for MUA must be supported by the following criteria:

   a. Past treatments have been exhausted but patient is a candidate for manipulative therapy and has responded favorably, but minimally.

   b. Sufficient care has been provided prior to recommending MUA (2-6 weeks).

   c. Manipulative procedures must have been tried in the clinical setting during this 2-6 week period of pre-MUA therapy.

   d. The patient's level of reproduced pain has begun to interfere with lifestyle (sleep, daily functional activities, work habits, etc.)

   e. Conditions being treated fall within the categories of those that have been recognized as responsive to MUA. The following conditions have responded with sufficient outcome to be classified as acceptable categories for application of the MUA procedure.

      (1) Patients whereby manipulation of the spine or other articulations is the treatment of choice; however, the patient's pain threshold will not allow the procedure to be performed.

      (2) Patients whereby manipulation of the spine or other articulations is the treatment of choice; however, due to the voluntary contraction of the supporting tissues and/or the splinting mechanism, patient treatment is delayed or may be prolonged. The MUA procedure may greatly shorten the time of treatment and may provide relief to the patient more rapidly.

      (3) Patients whereby manipulation of the spine or other articulations is the treatment of choice; however, due to the extent of the injury mechanism, conservative manipulation has not been effective in 2-6 weeks of care and a greater degree of movement to the affected joints is needed to be effective.

      (4) The patient is being considered for spinal disc surgery and the MUA procedure is an alternative or an interim step and may be used as a therapeutic and/or diagnostic tool in the overall consideration of the patient's condition.

      (5) Patients whereby manipulation of the spine or other articulations is the treatment of choice by the physician; however, due to the chronicity of the problem and/or fibrous tissue adhesions present, conservative manipulation is ineffective or would otherwise be ineffective.

2. **Diagnosis**

Each area treated must have a diagnosis. Statements of patient progress or response are combined to reveal the actual diagnosis that have been submitted for consideration of payment and/or have responded sufficiently as to be recognized as having valid response to MUA. Those diagnoses which have been shown to be most responsive include, but are not limited to, the following:

- Sclerotogenous pain medical branch of dorsal rami
- Cervical, thoracolumbar myofascial radiculitis
- IVD syndrome without fragmentation, sequestration, or significant osseous encroachment with or without radiculopathy
- Cervicobrachial pain syndrome from torticollis
- Chronic recurrent headache
- Failed back surgeries which do not involve hypermobile motion units and have been responsive to office clinical therapeutic trials
- Adhesive capsulitis relative to articular motion
- Paravertebral myofascial radicular muscle contracture related to functional biomechanical dysfunction syndromes (vertebral subluxation syndrome)

3. **Frequency and Follow-up**

Protocols for the number of MUA procedures should consider the following:

- Chronicity
- Length of current therapy program and progress as determined by progress protocols
- Patient age
- Number of previous injuries to same area
- Patient acceptance
- Muscle contracture level (beyond splinting)
- Level of intractable pain given 2-6 week protocol parameter
- Consideration of social life (interference with normal lifestyle)
- Response to the first MUA based on sound clinical documentation and protocols for determining patient progress
- Possible surgical intervention if procedure is not complete (meaning one might make patient a surgical candidate, two or three might alleviate the problem completely)
- Adhesion buildup from failed back surgery

Protocols for determining patient progress prior to and following the MUA:

Subjective Change

- Patient's pain index, visual analog scale
- Patient's ability to engage in active ROM
- Patient's change in daily routine activities
- Patient's change in job performance
- Patient's sleep habit changes and patterns
- Patient's dietary changes

Objective Change

- Change in measurable muscle mass
- Change in muscle contrcatability
- Change in EMG, NCV
- Change in muscle strength
- Change in controlled measurable passive ROM
- Change in radiographic studies(X-rays,CT,MRI)

4. **Safety**

The National Academy of MUA Physicians documents the need for a certified MUA physician.

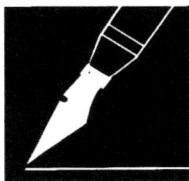

CHAPTER • FIFTEEN

AVERAGE CHIROPRACTIC TREATMENT FREQUENCY GUIDELINES

This is a general guide of typical frequency patterns seen in chiropractic. These are not meant to be an exact guide or a "cut off point," but to be used as a guide. They are derived from reasonable national utilization guidelines, current literature, and experience performing utilization reviews. These are only advisory in nature and should give you a general idea of typical treatment frequency parameters in the chiropractic profession.

Daily...1-2 Weeks (Must Be Clinically Justified)

4-5 Visits/Week ....1-2 Weeks (Must Be Clinically Justified)

3 Visits/Week ....Next 4-6 Weeks

2 Visits/Week ....Next 4-6 Weeks

1 Visit/Week ....Next 4-8 Weeks

2 Visits/Every 2 Weeks ....Next 4-8 Weeks

PEDIATRIC AND ADOLESCENT MANAGEMENT

Patient Age	Frequency	Duration
Up To 5 Years	4-8 Visits	4-6 Weeks
6-8 Years	6-10 Visits	4-8 Weeks
8-12 Years	10-14 Visits	5-9 Weeks
13-17 Years	12-18 Visits	6-12 Weeks
17-20 Years	16-24 Visits	8-14 Weeks
Over 21 Years	Adult Values	Adult Values

EXACERBATION'S AND REINJURY GUIDELINES
Note: The exacerbations must be properly documented in the patient's file.

Onset	Frequency	Duration
Mild Exacerbations or Reinjury	4-8 Visits	2-4 Weeks
Moderate Exacerbations or Reinjury	6-10 Visits	2-6 Weeks
Severe Exacerbations or Reinjury	12-20 Visits	4-8 Weeks

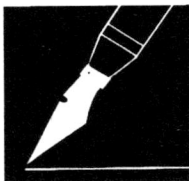

CHAPTER • SIXTEEN

"RED FLAGS"

The following is a partial list of criteria that may be used to identify those claims that are referred for utilization review. Each insurance company has their own set of standards that they use for guidelines. These are derived from personal communication with insurance industry personnel and experience performing utilization reviews. These include:

1. Excess charges. The treating facility is "unbundling" the reimbursement codes or the case has gone beyond a set threshold figure for cost.

2. Treatment continuing without documented reexaminations and a reduction in the treatment frequency.

3. Treatment is inconsistent with the diagnosis and multiple body areas are being treated. This would also include an embellished diagnosis or no diagnosis.

4. Treatment that does not start until several months after the date of injury or a case where there are several preexisting conditions.

5. Excessive diagnostic tests including several repeat x-ray examinations, especially when dealing with children.

6. Lengthy and prolonged treatment for the diagnosis "subluxation" in the absence of any other positive diagnostic testing.

7. "Unbundling" of treatment charges or billing for comprehensive visits for each date of service. The review would be directed toward the medical necessity of the level of service that was billed and to determine if the patient records supports the level of service that was billed and the medical decision making. A comprehensive visit in not medically necessary on each date of service. The comprehensive services would be restricted to initial and progress examinations if all of the components are found.

8. Continual use of passive therapies without a switch to active care.

9. Excessive or prolonged treatment when dealing with children.

10. Using more than 2 to 3 adjunctive modalities per visit with no reduction.

11. The insurance representative does not like chiropractors.

12. Treating doctor/clinic has a bad reputation. This may include prior questionable treatment patterns, questionable referrals to the same group of providers, or self referrals.

13. Multiple occupants injured in the same accident.

The person(s) determining which cases are sent for utilization review typically have no medical/chiropractic background. Claims representatives may send a case for review because or personal bias or ignorance. A case may also be reviewed because the claims examiner feels the patient should not be treating with a chiropractor for certain conditions, i.e. disc herniations, whiplash or children. We must understand that our profession comes under closer scrutiny than most other health care professions and we need to be prepared to deal with this accordingly.

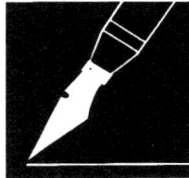

CHAPTER • SEVENTEEN

PROCEDURES WHICH ARE LIKELY TO TRIGGER A UTILIZATION REVIEW

This chapter details some of the more common procedures used in practice that may trigger a peer review. These procedures include clinical management protocols, billing practices, and questionable referrals. It is important to remember that using one of these procedures individually may not lead to a peer review but several of these procedures used in combination would likely lead to a review in most cases. Some of these procedures may be reasonable if there is a sufficient rationale for ordering the test or procedure.

1. **Unbundling of Examination or Treatment charges**

   An examination charge includes one fee for all of the elements of the examination including the chiropractic analysis, orthopedic and neurologic testing, range of motion, muscle testing, etc. "Unbundling" means that the treating doctor bills separately for one or more of the examination components, billing separately for the orthopedic/neurologic examination, consultation, muscle testing, and range of motion. Customary billing procedures include all of the elements of the examination. This may also include billing for an examination and adjustment on the same date of service without documentation indicating that both services did, in fact, take place. The examination charges also include the report of findings and the patient should not be billed separately for this. This may also include billing a higher level office visit than was actually performed.

2. **Extensive Daily Services**

   Under certain circumstances (for example, severe whiplash) the treating doctor may choose to initially treat the patient on a daily basis. This does not typically extend beyond one week. The documentation must support the clinical necessity of daily treatment. Daily treatment includes holidays, weekends, and the doctor's days off.

3. **X-ray Procedures**

   The typical billing procedure for x-rays includes one fee for both the professional and technical components. It is not accepted practice to bill separately for the taking of the x-rays and the interpretation of the x-rays unless the doctor is a DACBR, medical radiologist, or other qualified reading service.

Reading of x-rays taken at a different location can be billed under CPT code 76140 which is for a written report of x-rays taken elsewhere.

An x-ray series must include a minimum of two views at right angles of each other. Single view x-rays do not provide diagnostic information unless used in conjunction with a complete x-ray series. Single x-rays do not constitute a complete initial study. A single view can be taken within six weeks of when the initial study was performed. Initial x-rays should be directed at the area of complaint. Full spine x-rays should not be exposed unless there is clinical information supporting the use.

Sectional studies are always used for evaluation of trauma. Sectional studies offer less radiation exposure and greater clarity than full spine x-rays. Full spine x-rays are used to evaluate and monitor a scoliosis. A cervical spine series contains a minimum of three views: A-P, Lateral, and APOM. If foraminal encroachment is suspected or radicular involvement is present, right and left obliques may also be indicated. The Davis series is taken in the case of cervical spine trauma such as whiplash.

Routine thoracic x-rays include AP and Lateral views. P-A and lateral chest x-rays may also be included if the clinical information supports their use.

Routine lumbar x-rays include AP and lateral views. The L5/S1 spot view may be taken to view the lumbosacral junction. Oblique x-rays are not part of an initial study, but may be taken to further view the pars interarticularis. Clinical need must be established prior to the taking of flexion and extension views.

ACA guidelines for the use of oblique radiographs: "while there is little evidence to support routine acquisition of oblique radiographs of the lumbar spine, there is ample evidence to support acquisition of these views if the frontal and lateral views fail to adequately demonstrate therapeutically significant pathology which is clinically suspected, or where uncertainty exists about a reasonable potential for these diseases to be present."

Certain techniques within the chiropractic profession use repeat and post x-rays. These techniques include, but are not limited to, Pettibon, Grostic, and Spinal Biophysics. Repeat and post x-rays are judged by their ability to contribute to the therapeutic plan, differential diagnosis, and prognosis. One to two repeat x-ray studies are all that is usually utilized. Repeat x-rays are used for significant exacerbations or re-injuries, monitoring of a scoliosis or a fracture, and suspicion of advancing pathology. Providers must submit documentation supporting the use of repeat studies.

4. Substandard Documentation

Documentation is used to justify treatment/procedures rendered to third party payers. Inadequate records may have a role in triggering a utilization review. If a claims examiner is unsure whether the billings correlate with the treatment notes, he/she may be quicker to send the case for a utilization review. One of the most important points to case management is the use of progress examinations. Reevaluations are used to justify the continuation of treatment and to modify treatment according to the patient's progress or lack thereof.

5. **Excessive Diagnostic Testing**

The overuse of diagnostic procedures, especially those that are done in-office, will catch the eye of an experienced examiner. Diagnostic tests that are excessive, not indicated medically, or in areas other than the chief complaint, will draw the closest attention.

6. **Modality Utilization**

Several of the current guidelines indicate that the general rule of modality utilization is typically no more than two adjunctive modalities in addition to a spinal adjustment/office visit. In some instances (severe acute conditions), the use of three may be necessary for a short period of time but the desired benefit should be documented in the patient's file. The physiologic effects of the adjunctive modalities should not significantly overlap.

The usage of adjunctive modalities decreases as the patient progresses and there is a switch from passive to active care. Usually, no more than one adjunctive modality is used in addition to spinal adjustments during the final stage of treatment because active care is the treatment of choice.

7. **Diagnostic Imaging and Procedures**

Diagnostic tests must contribute to the differential diagnosis, prognosis, or therapeutic plan in order to meet the medical necessity criteria. (See Chapter 11 for the complete list of clinically necessary criteria). Referral for expensive tests such as MRI, CT, etc. may be subject to a utilization review. Review Chapter 11 for information about diagnostic imaging.

8. **Range of Motion Studies**

Billing separately for range-of-motion studies is typically not reasonable. These charges would be included as part of the examination or office visit. Under most circumstances, range of motion studies would not meet the criteria of medically necessary to be billed as a separate and distinct diagnostic testing procedure. However, if the range-of-motion studies were used as part of an impairment rating requested by an insurance carrier or an attorney, separate billing may be appropriate. Range-of-motion studies to be used as an outcome assessment should also not be billed as a separate and distinct procedure. These studies would be considered a "treatment management tool" and have no aid in contributing to a differential diagnosis.

9. **Concurrent Treatment**

Chiropractors routinely refer to other specialists during the course of normal case management. What is meant by concurrent treatment is that the patient is receiving the same or very similar treatment from two different providers at the same time. Examples would include treating with two chiropractors or having the same treatment done by both a chiropractor and a physical therapist. This may also include being treated by both a chiropractor and osteopath at the same time. I have reviewed cases where a patient was having similar treatment done by two doctors who have offices next to each other. The doctors under review have always denied that they knew there was concurrent treatment being rendered on the same dates of service.

10. **Manipulation Under Anesthesia**

This procedure is a very effective treatment for certain conditions. It is becoming more commonly utilized. The reason this procedure would be reviewed by an insurance carrier would be cost. Some insurance companies are still unfamiliar with MUA so they review it solely on cost or ignorance. The MUA criteria and protocols are found in Chapter 14. If you are using this procedure, you may want to contact the insurance carrier prior to performing MUA so that the carrier understands why you are doing it.

11. **Billing Joint Manipulation and Spinal Adjustment**

Billing for both spinal adjustments and joint mobilization in the same area on the same date would not constitute accepted practice. These would be considered a duplication of service since the spinal adjustment takes the joint through a greater range of motion than the joint mobilization.

12. **Durable Medical Goods**

The use of pillows, cushions, foot insoles, home rehabilitation equipment, and other supplies is often reasonable. Home TENS units, home spas, and mattresses may be subject to a utilization review. The reviewing doctor should apply the same medical necessity criteria to these supplies as he/she would to any other referral.

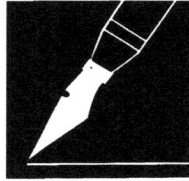

CHAPTER • EIGHTEEN

ETHICAL CONSIDERATIONS

This chapter is why I became involved in peer review. There seems to be a certain percentage of doctors performing reviews who have a reputation of unfairness. These doctors have been referred many cases with a very high percentage of these going in favor of the insurance carrier or requesting party. The reviewer gets rewarded by getting more referrals, the review company is happy because the insurance carrier sends them more work, and the insurance carrier sees the case end. It becomes a vicious cycle.

Do not allow yourself to be swayed or influenced by insurance adjusters or review company personnel in making your determination. Never change your opinions when the report is finalized. I have been asked to change my opinions. When I declined, I was sent no future work. You must be prepared for this scenario and conduct yourself according to the ethical standards found below.

Reviewing clinicians must always adhere to strict ethical guidelines when performing a review. The reviewer must at all times act like a referee when giving a determination regarding a particular matter. This means that the reviewer must never take sides or allow themselves to lose their ability to be objective when rendering a decision. A reviewer must never receive payment contingent upon their review decisions nor should they be influenced by the requesting party in any manner. Reviewers must be aware that rendering an opinion contrary to what the requesting party would like may result in no future work being sent by that requesting party.

The reviewer must protect the confidentiality of a patient's condition and should not discuss the practices of their colleagues. Reviewers must always respect their colleagues, the patient, and the other parties involved in the review process. If a reviewer is unable to render an objective opinion for a particular reason, he/she should decline the case. Examples may include performing a review on a close friend or a former patient who is currently treating with another doctor.

Reviewers must be consistent in their determinations and should never hold other providers to higher standards than they hold themselves. The promotion of their profession and the responsibility to the patient, attending doctor or clinician, and review organization must always be considered. The reviewer should always charge a reasonable fee and perform the review in a timely manner.

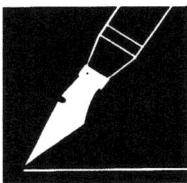

CHAPTER • NINETEEN

PHONE CONSULTATION GUIDELINES

Phone consultations are part of certain reviews. The phone consultation can be a challenge depending on the demeanor and attitude of both the reviewer and clinician. Both the reviewer and attending clinician must exercise professionalism and cordiality. The reviewer should always try to arrange a time that is mutually convenient in advance of a phone consultation. This will assure that both parties will have sufficient time (typically 15 minutes) to discuss the clinical aspects of the case at hand. It is recommended that the conversation be limited to the case under review and never get into a conversation about the current literature or the qualifications of the reviewer or practitioner. You should make at least three attempts on different days and document these attempts.

The reviewer should correlate the information gathered during the phone conversation with the information in the medical file in order to determine the accuracy of the information. For this reason, the reviewer should never reveal his/her determinations during the phone conversation. The reviewer should also not be intimidated by the treating clinician into making a decision in favor of the provider under review.

The phone conversation may be terminated if the provider under review does not limit his/her comments and conversation to the case that is under review. Reasonable language is always expected of both parties and may also be grounds to terminate the phone conversation. If one of the parties wishes to go "off the record," this should be identified. The details of the phone conversation should be accurately depicted in the peer report and both parties should take notes about what was discussed.

The reviewer should ask questions regarding the current clinical status such as the subjective and objective findings, current treatment including frequency, limitations in activities of daily living, documented exacerbations, re-injuries or new injuries, complicating factors and/or preexisting conditions, estimate of future care, concurrent treatment, evaluations with specialists, diagnostic imaging, diagnosis, and estimate of when maximum medical improvement will be attained.

The purpose of the phone consultation is to discuss the clinical aspects of the case under review and to allow the provider to give verbal input regarding the case. The topic of the phone consultation is not the medical literature, personal beliefs, etc. The topic is the patient and the case under review. Both parties should keep notes of what was discussed and at least three attempts on different days should be made by the reviewing doctor.

EXAMPLE

The following represents an example of a phone consultation. Dr. Smith is the treating doctor and Dr. Jones is the reviewer. Each phone consultation will vary somewhat depending on the specifics of each case but this should give you a general idea of how a phone consultation should be conducted.

Dr. Jones: Hello Dr. Smith. My name is Dr. Jones. I am conducting a utilization review on a patient of yours, Ms. Jenny Lumbago. I am calling as you requested to discuss the clinical aspects of the case before I render a final determination. I have a few questions. The last date of service I have is 2/3/97, have you seen Ms. Lumbago since then?

Dr. Smith: Yes. I saw Ms. Lumbago on 2/10, 2/17, and 2/24.

Dr. Jones: So the current frequency of treatment is weekly?

Dr. Smith: Yes.

Dr. Jones: What treatment are you currently doing on Ms. Lumbago?

Dr. Smith: Spinal adjustments, muscle stimulation, and a home rehabilitation protocol.

Dr. Jones: What are Ms. Lumbago's current subjective and objective findings?

Dr. Smith: Her low back pain is much improved. She only has mild discomfort and is tolerating the exercise protocol well. Her range of motion, reflexes, and straight leg raising test are all improved.

Dr. Jones: Are there any complicating factors in the history or examination?

Dr. Smith: Ms. Lumbago had lumbar spine surgery two years ago and she is also diabetic.

Dr. Jones: What are your expectations for MMI and expectation for future care.

Dr. Smith: I will be releasing Ms. Lumbago in two weeks unless she suffers an exacerbation. Any future treatment will be on a PRN basis for symptomatic exacerbations.

Dr. Jones: Do you have anything further you would like to add?

Dr. Smith: No.

Dr. Jones: Thank you, Dr. Smith. I will review the file again and render my determination. Have a nice day!

Dr. Smith: Thank You!

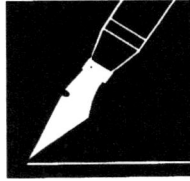

CHAPTER • TWENTY

REPORT WRITING FORMAT

Writing a peer report is a skill in itself. One must not only be able to make decisions about a case, but also the reviewer must be able to clearly and concisely relate these opinions to other parties. You must always remember that several people will read the reports and that most of them may have no medical background. These people include insurance representatives, attorneys, and the patients themselves.

There are six different areas to a peer report:

1. *General Information*

   Date of Review:

   Patient Name:

   SS#:

   Date of Injury:

   Review# or Claim#:

   To Whom It May Concern:

   I have reviewed the medical records provided on the above-mentioned case for the purpose of a retrospective review. The following opinions are based solely upon submitted records which are listed below, absent the opportunity to personally examine the patient. Final benefit determinations are the sole responsibility of the insurance carrier.

2. *Records Reviewed* (Example)
   - UR assignment
   - UR request
   - Lillard Chiropractic
   - Initial history and examination 1/1/96
   - Progress notes 1/1/96-4/6/96
   - Case history 1/1/96
   - Joe Orthopod
   - Examination 2/2/96

3. *Case Review/Summary*

Summarize the records that you have reviewed. Indicate the mechanism of injury and whether any emergency treatment was received.

Summarize any treatment rendered prior to chiropractic care and include the type of treatment and response to care.

Include pertinent information from specialists consulted. Make sure to include the clinical impression and recommendations. Also include a summary of any diagnostic tests and their findings.

Explain the treatment frequency, number of visits, and response to care of the chiropractic treatment under review.

4. *Phone consultations*

This paragraph details the information that was gathered during the phone conversation.

5. *Clinical Opinion/Utilization Review Decisions*

Answer all of the questions that the requesting party has asked. Give a clear and concise answer as well as a rationale to support you opinion.

6. *Closure*

It is common practice to add a closure or "disclaimer" to your reports. The following is an example:

The opinions rendered in this case are the opinions of the reviewer. This review has been conducted without a medical examination of the individual reviewed. This review is based on documents provided to us by the provider with the assumption that the diagnosis is true and correct. This report is a clinical assessment and opinion conducted with the information available. It does not constitute per se recommendation for specific claims to be made or enforced.

QUESTIONS THAT MAY BE ASKED:

1. Based upon submitted documentation, in your opinion, what injuries were substantiated as being sustained on the date of loss?
2. Does the medical documentation substantiate the medical necessity and appropriateness of care rendered?
3. Usual and customary length of treatment?
4. Has the maximum level of therapeutic benefit been achieved?
5. Comment on the medical necessity or past, present, and future treatment?
6. Comment on the reasonable and necessity or treatment?

Reviewers may be asked to comment on issues such as the diagnosis, referral for diagnostic procedures, referral for specialty consultations, impairment ratings, home TENS units, etc.

Be sure to proofread your report to make sure you have commented on all of the issues that were raised. You should always strive for accuracy and completeness when rendering an opinion on a particular matter.

If you are reviewing records as an "in house" consultant for an insurance company, you may not even be required to render a written report. You should, however, outline important aspects of the case for future reference, if needed.

WHAT IS AN INITIAL DETERMINATION?

An initial determination is the first step in the review process in most instances. This is the first review to be done on a particular. The term "initial" implies that there is another review that may potentially follow it. This second review, which is sometimes an appeal of the first review, is called a reconsideration.

WHAT IS A RECONSIDERATION?

A reconsideration is a second review that is requested after the initial determination, and the review covers the same treatment and treatment dates as the initial determination. The purpose is to "reconsider" the opinions of the initial reviewer. These can usually be requested by any party involved in the review during a specified time frame after the initial review determination is put into effect. In Pennsylvania, you have 30 days to request a reconsideration under the automobile law.

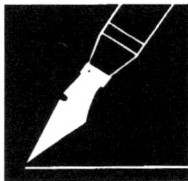

CHAPTER • TWENTY-ONE

X-RAY REPORT WRITING

There are four components to a radiology report:

1. *Patient and view identification-patient name, age, and sex.* Date of the exam and date of the report. Where x-rays were taken if different from your office. Views-what areas were x-rayed.

    Example: Patient:

    Date of Examination:

    Date of report:

    Age:

    Sex:

    Views: Cervical spine: A-P, APOM, left lateral (example)

2. *Findings:* A description of what appears on the radiological report. The most important finding should be done first with different features being separated by paragraphs.

    A: Alignment

    B: Bone

    C: Cartilage

    S: Soft tissue

    Example: The cervical spine is hypolordotic. There are early degenerative changes in the mid to lower cervical spine consisting of loss of disc height and osteophyte formation. Osseous density is adequate.

3. *Impressions:* A list of diagnosis with differentials based on the findings. List in same order as in "findings."

    Example: 1. Degenerative changes of the cervical spine.

    2. Hypolordotic cervical spine.

4. *Recommendations:* Might include suggestions on additional radiographic, laboratory, and clinical examinations. Treatment recommendations are not usually found here.

    Example: 1. Flexion and extension studies of the cervical spine.

Remember that all areas in the collimated beam must be accounted for and make sure the study is complete(minimum of two views at right angles). If there is no report, did the service, in fact, take place?

SELECTED RADIOLOGY TERMINOLOGY

Trauma
- Compression, fracture, callus, alignment, spondylysis

Congenital
- Developemental, dysplasia, sacralization, lumbarization, agenesis

Arthridites
- Arthrosis, degenerative joint disease, degenerative disc disease, sclerosis, spurring, end plate, joint space, spondyloarthropathy, osteophytes, intervertebral, spondylosis, syndesmophytes

Infection
- Periosteal elevation, involucrum, lysis

Biomechanics
- Curvature, hyperkyphosis, hypokyphosis, scoliosis, pelvic unleveling, instability, subluxation, hyperlordosis, hypolordosis, hypermobility, hypomobility

Soft Tissue
- Calcification, calcific, calculi, artherosclerotic plaquing

SAMPLE X-RAY REPORT 1

Doctor:	Francis Smith, D.C.	Patient:	James Taylor
Date of Examination:	1/1/90	Age:	62
Date of Report:	1/1/90	Sex:	Male

Cervical Spine:

A-P, lateral, open-mouth, flexion, extension, right and left oblique projections reveals loss of cervical lordosis with some degree of hyperflexion of C3 on C4. The disc spaces appear well maintained. The flexion and extension studies reveal questionable segmental hypermobility of C4 on C5, especially on extension.

IMPRESSIONS

1. Loss of cervical lordosis with hyperflexion malposition of C3 on C4.

RECOMMENDATIONS

1. Follow-up as clinically indicated.

Gregg J. Fisher, D.C.

SAMPLE X-RAY REPORT 2

PATIENT: Sam Smith

AGE: 73

SEX: Male

DATE OF X-RAYS: January 25, 1997

DATE OF REPORT: January 25, 1997

Cervical Spine: A-P, Lateral, A-P Open Mouth; Thoracic spine: A-P, Lateral; Lumbar Spine: A-P, Lateral.

There is pelvic unleveling low on the left with a mild right convex lumbar curve. There is no evidence of recent fracture or dislocation. There is a healed compression deformity of the L1 vertebral body. There is also a considerable amount of loss of disc height and osteophyte formation at the T12/L1 and L2/L3 motion units.

There is a moderate degree of degenerative changes seen throughout the cervical spine consisting of loss of disc height and osteophyte formation most evident at C5/C6 with apparent interbody fusion.

The thoracic spine is unremarkable.

IMPRESSIONS:

1. Healed compression deformity of L1.
2. Moderate to advanced degenerative changes in the cervical and lumbar spines as described above.

RECOMMENDATIONS:

1. Flexion/extension studies of the cervical spine to evaluate ligamentous integrity.

Gregg J. Fisher, D.C.

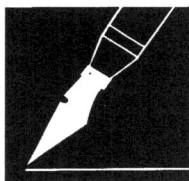

CHAPTER • TWENTY-TWO

INDEPENDENT EXAMINATIONS

Independent examinations use an "unbiased" examiner to render an opinion regarding a particular patient and injury or circumstance. Independent examinations are done by someone other than the treating doctor. The are typically asked for by insurance companies and attorneys. The examiner may also choose to testify for the requesting party if he/she desires. The independent examination includes both a records review and a physical examination.

The independent exam is thought to allow someone who has no personal attachment with the patient render an opinion. It would be advisable to have an office assistant accompany you in the examination room to avoid any allegations of misconduct. It is also advisable not to allow recording devices in the room when an examination is being done.

A friend or relative may accompany the patient, but they should not participate in the exam or "coach" the patient in any manner. If they attempt to do so, it would be appropriate to document this in your report and ask the person to leave the examination room.

SUGGESTED IME FORMAT

GENERAL INFORMATION

Include the date of the report and information such as the claim number, patient name, and date of injury.

OPENING PARAGRAPH

Include a few sentences to describe the date and time the examination took place, and physical description of the patient including observations. Details of any particulars of the examination are also helpful.

Example:

This 69-year-old white female was referred by II opinion, Inc., 4423 N. Front St., Harrisburg, PA 17110, for an independent medical examination on April 27, 1995 for injuries apparently the result of an automobile accident on June 10, 1993. She is presently being treated by Harvey Lumbago DC, 1313 Luck Lane, Williamsport, PA 17703.

HISTORY OF INJURY

This section should contain a brief history of how the accident occurred. The types of vehicles involved and damage should be noted. Was the seatbelt being worn? Was the impact anticipated? Did cars have to be towed?

Example:

Mrs. Clinton stated that on 6/10/93 she was driving her 1980 Cadillac and was stopped to make a left-hand turn. She was struck from behind by a Subaru station wagon. "She pushed me I don't know how many feet." She stated she was wearing her seatbelt and did not anticipate the accident. Mrs. Clinton stated that there was about $1,000 worth of damage done to her car and that the other car had to be towed due to the front end damage.

PAST MEDICAL HISTORY

This section should include significant past medical history as related by the patient's surgeries, medications, work history, and any past medical conditions that would be pertinent to this patient's situation. Chiropractic care previous to the accident and previous injuries or conditions are important.

Example:

Mrs. Clinton's past medical history includes treatment for heart disease and a stomach ulcer. Her surgeries include angioplasty in 1990 and bowel obstruction approximately 45 years ago. Current medications include Zantac, Toprol, and Flurosemide. Mrs. Clinton is single and smokes 1 pack of cigarettes per day. She retired in 1990 and past occupations include waitress, bookkeeper, and sales. She has had previous chiropractic care but none for several years before the accident. She states she likes to read in bed. She denies ever having injured her cervical spine or being treated for neck pain prior to 6/10/93.

PRESENT COMPLAINTS

A detailed description of the patient's current complaints relating to the accident or injury should be included if the patient feels improved under the current treatment.

Example:

Mrs. Clinton stated that after the accident on 6/10/93 she was "upset, shaking, and began to experience a headache." The next day she states she woke up in pain so she looked through the phone book and saw Dr. Lumbago's ad. She complains of constant neck pain that varies in intensity. She points to the mid-lower cervical spine as the location of the pain and also states she has pain in her right and left upper trapezius. She also has pain that radiates to the mid and lower back. She states she has headaches but is unable to determine the frequency. She states she has loss of grip strength when lifting and grasping certain objects. She states she cannot do housework such as vacuuming, cleaning, and wiping the floor without becoming aggravated. She states she gets relief while lying on the couch using a moist heating pad. Generally speaking, rest helps and activity aggravates her.

Mrs. Clinton is being currently treated by Dr. Lumbago. She is being treated once every two weeks. She states she has been doing this since October or November. She states Dr. Lillard calls this "maintenance care." She states she gets slight relief but this depends on her activities. When asked if she feels better since starting treatment with Dr. Lillard, she could only respond "I think so."

Mrs. Clinton was also seen by Dr. X who prescribed a course of physical therapy but states "the insurance would only allow so long." She was told by Dr. X that "she will have to learn to live with it."

PHYSICAL EXAMINATION

General appearance and attitude. Vitals signs and how they moved around the room, walked, etc. Complete cervical, thoracic, and lumbar spine examinations as applicable. The examining doctor should focus in on the area of complaint. Malingering and special orthopedic tests would be done here.

Example:

Mrs. Clinton appears well-oriented, pleasant, but somewhat nervous. She holds her head in slight forward flexion. She was able to move on and off the examination table without difficulty. Blood pressure was 130/80. Pulse was 80 beats per minute and respiration was 16 breaths per minute.

Cervical spine examination revealed the following: Active cervical ROM was decreased in all ranges, especially extension and right and left lateral flexion. Motion did increase during doctor-assisted passive motion. She experienced pain on resisted right and left lateral flexion. There was tenderness in the cervical spine and joint fixation in the mid to lower cervical spine. Upper extremity reflexes were +1/4 bilaterally. She did show weakness of the right wrist flexor extensor on motor examination being graded +4/5. Mensuration revealed no atrophy. Spurling's, Bakody, Dejerine, Adson's, Eden's, and Wright's tests were all negative bilaterally. Liebman's test was positive to slight pressure. Simulated grip strength test was positive.

Lumbosacral examination revealed the following: ROM was decreased with no pain. There was no pain on resisted ROM. Sensory, motor, reflex, and mensuration revealed no abnormalities. Bechterew's, SLR, Nachlas, Femoral Stretch, Hibb's, and Sacroiliac Extension tests were negative bilaterally. There was tenderness in the right sacroiliac region.

REVIEW OF RECORDS

This section should address all of the records reviewed. If you are viewing x-rays, make sure to comment on quality and completeness of the study. Summarize all previous treatment and results. Make sure to list previous diagnoses. List all diagnostic tests and pertinent findings. List key points from other physician records. Since you may be examining a patient months or years after an injury, the records review will be a very important component of the independent examination. List all of the records reviewed and summarize. Comment on gaps in treatment, frequency of reevaluations, and daily progress notes.

Example:

In a report dated 1/23/95, Dr. Lumbago recommends care at the frequency of 1-2 times per week and calls this supportive in nature. This report also states that chiropractic care only provides temporary relief and that Mrs. Clinton "shows a spontaneous return of these symptoms with normal activities of daily living."

You may be given the original x-rays to look at. Examine them as you would normally and do a brief description. Make sure to comment on quality of the films, completeness of the study and any artifacts or significant pathology.

IMPRESSION

This section should include the impression and diagnosis of the examining physician. Include inconsistencies in the examination and/or conclusions of the attending doctor in the context of your discussion.

NEED FOR CONTINUED TREATMENT

This section should address the examining physician's feelings regarding the need and recommendations for continued treatment.

DISCUSSION

This section will include comments regarding the examination, records review, and what your opinions regarding the patient are.

Example:

Mrs. Clinton stated that prior to the MVA she was asymptomatic. Since the accident she complains of increased symptoms with her ADLs. Her examination findings seem to correlate with her diagnostic studies.

Dr. Lumbago stated that Mrs. Clinton has decreased grip strength. During simulated grip strength testing she was able to hold my hands firmly and when I attempted to pull away, she gripped even tighter before she realized what she was doing.

It appears that the MVA activated Mrs. Clinton's preexisting degenerative changes, causing them to become symptomatic expressive. The report dated 9/23/93 calls this a serious and permanent injury. The degeneration itself would be considered permanent in nature.

Mrs. Clinton is experiencing symptoms in her cervical spine. The magnitude of these symptoms is unclear. One must question why she would require treatment on a regular basis for the rest of her life when she is able to travel by car to North Carolina and Florida for three months and only be treated for one week during this time frame.

PROGNOSIS

This section should address the prognosis of the patient depending on the examination, records review, and impression of the examining physician. If the patient has not reached MMI and the requesting party asks you to address MMI, it is appropriate to state that the patient has not reached MMI and that a future examination may be needed to address maximum improvement.

If you feel the patient needs to be examined by another professional then state this in your report. It is important to make these recommendations especially when you may have found or suspect a condition the treating doctor has overlooked.

Example:

Due to the degeneration in the cervical spine, it is possible Mrs. Clinton may experience symptoms indefinitely. Mrs. Clinton has reached maximum improvement for her injuries and no further regularly scheduled treatment would result in a clinical progression of her condition.

RETURN TO WORK

This section should address the impressions of the examining physician in regards to the patient's return to work status. Include documentation of physical capacities evaluation form with the report.

IME SAMPLE

August 12, 1995

Mrs. Jill Brown
Claims Representative
Your Ins. Co.

RE: Charles Chan
Claim: 111222
DOL: 6/24/94

Dear Mrs. Brown,

This 21 year old Asian male was referred by Your Ins. Co. for an independent examination on August 10, 1995 for injuries apparently the result of an automobile accident on June 26, 1994. He is presently being treated by Tom Toggle, D.C., 110 Main St., Mytown, PA 10000.

HISTORY OF INJURY

Mr. Chan stated that on 6/24/94 he was driving his 1987 S10 pickup when he was stopped at a red light. He was struck from behind by another car described as a S10 Blazer. At the time of the accident, Mr. Chan reported to be "eating a cupcake" and not wearing his seatbelt. He was also reported to hit his head on the steering wheel and was temporarily knocked unconscious. Mr. Chan stated that the other vehicle was towed due to front end damage and the police were called. There was over $2,900 damage done to Mr. Chan's truck.

PAST MEDICAL HISTORY

Mr. Chan's medical history is unremarkable for illness or disease. He does not smoke or drink and reports being in good health. He denies ever having had surgery. He denies neck or back pain prior to the accident on 6/24/94. The only medication reported was Tylenol. Prior to the accident, he was working as a "cutter" in a clothing factory. He had worked there three months prior to the accident. He also works "a few hours on the weekend" at his family's restaurant.

PRESENT COMPLAINTS

Mr. Chan stated that his neck pain started one to two hours after the accident. He points to the right upper cervical region as the location of the pain. He states "it pulls once in a while." He states the pain is intermittent and can "grab." Mr. Chan states Tylenol and moist heat give him some relief when he has pain. He states he can go several days without pain. Treatment prior to chiropractic care included muscle relaxers and a short course of physical therapy.

Page 2
RE: C. Chan

He states that Dr. Toggle's treatment has helped somewhat and he is currently being treated from one visit every two weeks to two times a week depending on how he feels. I asked Mr. Chan why he is seeing two chiropractors at once and he stated he doesn't like to wait so he goes to the office that isn't as busy.

He also describes low back pain that he says started two days after the accident. He describes the pain as mild and episodic. Mr. Chan relates morning stiffness approximately one time per month.

EXAMINATION

Mr. Chan appears well-oriented, pleasant, and cooperative. His gait is unremarkable and he moves on and off the examination table without difficulty. Blood pressure is 120/80, pulse is 72 beats per minute, and respiration is 16 breaths per minute.

Cervical spine examination revealed the following: All active ranges of motion were within normal limits except a slight decrease in right rotation. All passive ranges of motion were within normal limits and produced no pain. There was no pain on resisted motion. Motor, reflex, sensory, and mensuration revealed no abnormalities in the upper extremities bilaterally. Adson's, Eden's, Wright's, Shoulder Depressor, and Spurling's were all negative bilaterally. There was slight local pain in the upper cervical spine produced on Spurling's test. There were no trigger points or spasm in the cervicothoracic paraspinal musculature or upper trapezii. Leibman's test produced excruciating pain to light pressure indicating a low pain threshold.

Lumbosacral examination revealed the following: Ranges of motion within normal limits with no pain. There was no pain on resisted motion. Motor, reflex, sensory, and mensuration revealed no abnormalities in the lower extremities bilaterally. Straight leg raising test was negative to 70 degrees. Valsalva, Bechterew, Sacro-iliac Extension, Nachlas, Femoral Stretch, and Fabere were negative bilaterally. Burns Bench test was positive suggesting malingering.

REVIEW OF RECORDS:

- ER records and billings from Hospital
- Cervical spine x-ray report 6/26/94
- Jim Walker DC:
  - Case History 7/20/94
  - 3 pages of progress notes showing services 7/20/94-3/3/95.
  - 22 HCFA forms
- Tom Toggle, D.C.
  - PI questionnaire, undated
  - 2 pages of progress notes showing dates of service 8/8/94-11/16/94
  - 7-page narrative to attorney, 3/1/95

Page 3
RE: C. Chan

The records provided for review indicate that Mr. Chan was seen at the hospital on 6/26/94. He was x-rayed, diagnosed with a "neck strain," prescribed a soft collar, medication, and released. He subsequently had three sessions of physical therapy and was released on 7/12/94 "feeling much better."

Mr. Chan consulted Dr. Walker on 7/20/94. treatment consisted of adjustments, hot packs, and intersegmental traction. There was no examination, diagnosis, treatment plan, or reevaluations provided for review.

Dr. Toggle was consulted on 8/8/94. There was no examination, diagnosis, or history taken. Progress notes were minimal. I gathered most of my information from the seven-page narrative to Mr. Chan's attorney. Dr. Toggle states that x-rays taken at his office show "permanent soft tissue damage" and "indicate and unstable cervical situation."

X-RAY EXAMINATION

The insurance carrier requested that I x-ray Mr. Chan. Cervical spine A-P, lateral, A-P open mouth, flexion, and extension views were taken. These revealed a well-maintained cervical spine and were unremarkable.

DISCUSSION

There are many inconsistencies in this case. Mr. Chan was able to fully turn his head on Adson's test but when I was doing range-of-motion he complained of pain and had decreased motion. He also refused to do Burns Bench test saying he couldn't do it.

Dr. Toggle would not release his x-rays for this examination. His report to Mr. Chan's attorney states that there is "an unstable cervical situation." However, the x-rays I took show a very well-maintained cervical spine.

Mr. Chan does have some minor joint dysfunction in his cervical spine. This may have several causes and would not necessarily be due to the automobile accident. Under proper care, this problem would resolve in a short period of time.

I feel Mr. Chan's injuries from the automobile accident are well-healed. He has no residual problems and is capable of full employment. I feel that he has some psychological overlay at the present time.

WORK RECOMMENDATION

There are no work restrictions.

FUTURE TREATMENT RECOMMENDATIONS

I do not feel that any regularly scheduled chiropractic treatment at this time would be necessary. Mr. Chan may need counseling to get back to his normal activities.

Page 4
RE: C. Chan

RECOMMENDATIONS

I would strongly urge the carrier to acquire the x-rays taken by Dr. Toggle for analysis and comparison to those taken here in my office.

If I can be of further assistance, please feel free to contact me.

Sincerely,

Gregg Fisher, D.C.

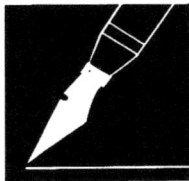

CHAPTER • TWENTY-THREE

MEDICO-LEGAL PREPARATION

DEPOSITION

An out-of-court examination of a witness, under oath, before a court reporter. Same as testimony given at trial but with no judge or jury. Lawyers question the witness concerning any matters which can be admitted at trial.

HOW IS DEPOSITION USED?

1. *Evidence at trial:* May be used as evidence at trial.
2. *Discovery:* May be used to help discover leads for evidence or facts that may be used at trial.
3. *Impeachment of witness:* May be used to discredit a witness at trial if it varies from their deposition testimony.
4. *Review of the witness:* A deposition gives attorneys the opportunity to evaluate a witness.

DO'S AND DON'TS FOR THE MEDICAL WITNESSES

The law department of the AMA formulated a useful guide for doctors to follow in the preparation and presentation of their testimony in the courtroom. These rules were published in the AMA Proceedings of the National Medicolegal Symposium held on November 8 and 9, 1963, pp. 227-229.

1. Do take the role of the medical witness seriously. Your function is of prime importance in the administration of justice.
2. Don't agree to or accept compensation for your services contingent upon the outcome of the litigation. This practice is unethical and can tend to destroy the value of your testimony if exposed.
3. Do insist on full preparation for your testimony with the attorney.
4. Don't act as an advocate or partisan in the trial of the case.
5. Do be as thorough as possible in examining a patient in preparation for trial.
6. Don't exaggerate.
7. Do inform the attorney who calls you as a witness of all unfavorable as well as favorable information developed by your examination.
8. Don't try to bluff. If you don't know the answer, don't guess.
9. Do be frank concerning your financial arrangements about testifying.

10. Don't regard it as an admission of ignorance to indicate that your opinion is not absolutely conclusive. You are testifying with a reasonable degree of medical certainty, not an absolutely conclusive degree of certainty.

11. Do answer all questions honestly and frankly. Reluctance or withholding may tend to discredit your testimony.

12. Don't use technical terminology which may not be understood.

13. Do be willing to disagree with so-called authorities if you believe they are wrong. Give sound reasons for your disagreement.

14. Don't be smug. A modest attitude will be apt to elicit a more favorable response.

15. Do be courteous despite any provocation.

16. Don't lose your temper.

17. Do pause briefly before answering questions on cross-examination to give the attorney an opportunity to object if he desires.

18. Don't allow yourself to be forced into a "yes" or "no" answer if a qualified answer is required. You have a right to explain or qualify your answer if necessary for a truthful response.

The key to any expert witness testimony is preparation. As an expert, you should be aware of the strengths and weaknesses of any case you are testifying about. The opposing attorney will try to discredit your testimony based upon weaknesses in your record keeping and case management. You may also choose to write your own direct examination questions and write cross-examination questions for the opposing expert witnesses. The opposing attorney may attack your qualifications, ask you questions about anatomy, or be hostile toward chiropractors.

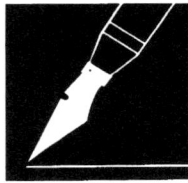

CHAPTER • TWENTY-FOUR

RECORD KEEPING EXAMPLES WITH CRITIQUE

In this chapter, we will show several examples of record keeping. This includes examples of SOAP notes, initial histories, reexaminations, adjunctive procedure notes, etc. At the end of the chapter, there will be a short critique for each example.

EXAMPLE 1

History: The patient states that he was involved in an automobile accident on 11/4/95. He was the belted driver of a pickup that was traveling in the left lane of traffic. A car in the right lane make a sudden lane change hitting the patient's car on the right side. He states he was jerked forward and that a jack behind the seat hit him in the back. He points to the left dorsolumbar area as the location of the problem. He was treated in the ER at Evangelical Hospital after the accident. He was x-rayed and diagnosed as being "bruised." He has tried home medication in the form of Advil with some relief. "I've been trying to live with the pain but it keeps getting worse." He denies radiating pain or pain with respiration. He states the pain is gradually getting worse and is increased with activity. Lying on his back increases the pain.

EXAMPLE 2

History: The patient presents with a continued complaint of low back pain. She states "it is sore around my beltline and into my right hip." She feels improved under our care rating her pain a 4 on a scale of 1 to 10, with 1 being minimal pain and 10 being severe pain. She describes intermittent "burning" in her right foot. She states her low back pain is worse after standing for long periods of time. She states bending forward increases her pain. She has used cryotherapy at home as directed and flexibility exercises. Her job entails lifting, bending, twisting, and climbing a ladder.

Examination: Lower extremity ROM is decreased. Lower extremity motor is +4/5 right and +5/5 left. Lower extremity reflexes are +2/4 bilaterally and lower extremity sensory is intact. SLR is positive on the right at 50 degrees with pain at L4/5 to right leg. Braggard's test increases the pain. WLR and Fajersztajn's tests are negative. Valsalva's maneuver produces localized pain at L4/5. There is joint fixation at L4/5. There are trigger points in the right sacrospinalis and right gluteus. Sacroiliac extension test is positive on the right and negative on the left.

Assessment: Traumatic exacerbation of bulging disc at L4/5 is improving. Cervical, lumbar, and sacroiliac segmental dysfunction. Possible right lower extremity radicular symptoms.

Discussion: Treatment will consist of spinal adjustments and myofascial release at the frequency of two times a week for four weeks at which time the patient will be reevaluated. She will continue her home exercise and home therapies. She should not work for two weeks. I would like to start the Backsys protocol in a few weeks.

EXAMPLE 3

8/14/95	Neck pain C5 PRS	9/5/95	C5 PRS
8/18/95	C2 PLS	9/8/95	C2 PLS
8/21/95	C5 PRS	9/14/95	C5 Getting Better
8/24/95	Home moist heat	9/18/95	C5
8/29/95	C5 PRS	9/21/95	C5
9/2/95	C5	9/24/95	Exercises.

EXAMPLE 4

9/12/94	ASLA Back feels great.
9/18/94	Failed appt.
9/24/94	Failed appt.
9/28/94	ASLA 3 wks.
10/12/94	Failed appt.
10/15/94	Failed appt.
10/17/94	ASLA 3 wks.
11/7/94	ASLA Headache 3 wks.

EXAMPLE 5

2/29/95

S: Patient presents today and states "I am not real bad today." Patient states that she has had a decrease in her upper back and shoulder area discomfort over the last week. Patient states she still does have some discomfort and points to the right and left upper trapezius and the upper thoracic spine as the location of the pain. Patient denies distal or radiating signs and symptoms.

Patient also states that she is improved in her lower back. Patient states that the pain in her lumbosacral spine is intermittent and has been improved over the last 1-2 days.

O: Straight leg raising test, Hibbs, and Fabere are negative right and left. There is a trigger point in the left gluteus maximus. There is joint fixation and tenderness at 2 and 3D. There are trigger points in the right and left upper trapezius.

A: Patient is improved.

P: A cervical pillow was discussed with the patient today and I feel that this would be beneficial to treat her problem. Patient has been instructed to return in 10 days.

1/10/96

S: Patient presents today and states "I woke up with a lot of pain." Patient complains that she has had cervico-thoracic area pain that has been increased since last week. Patient states that she wanted to get in here for a treatment but due to all the snow she could not get in as planned. Patient points to the lower cervical and upper thoracic spine as the location of the pain.

O: There is joint fixation and tenderness at 5/6C and 2 and 3D. There are trigger points in the right and left upper trapezius. Straight leg raising test is negative right and left. Sacroiliac extension test is negative right and positive left with pain in the left sacroiliac and gluteus region. There are trigger points in the left gluteus region.

A: Patient is somewhat regressed since last visit.

P: Patient has been instructed to return in 10 days and use home moist heat.

EXAMPLE 6

Dec 29 1995   COMMENTS:

Trt Codes   <u>S:</u>   CERVICAL ✓ DORSAL ✓ LUMBO-PELVIC <u>Jan 16 1996</u> _____
_____   <u>O:</u>   spasm C:_____ D:_____L: tender C:____D:____L:____ _____
99215   <u>A:</u>   <u>improving</u>   unchanged   regressing   temp. relief   _____
97260   <u>P:</u>   <u>reschedule in</u>_____days weeks months   _____
_____   Exam EMS heat diathermy traction massage ultrasound ice   _____
_____   adjustment: C   D   L ✓   P ✓   extremity   _____
_____   Single   ✓   ✓   ✓   ✓   ____   _____
                          multiple ✓   ____ ____ ____ ____   _____

Jan 03 1996   COMMENTS:

Trt Codes   <u>S:</u>   CERVICAL ✓ DORSAL ✓ LUMBO-PELVIC ✓ _____
_____   <u>O:</u>   spasm C:_____ D:_____L: tender C:✓ D:✓ L:✓ _____
97260   <u>A:</u>   improving   unchanged   <u>regressing</u>   temp. relief   _____
97014   <u>P:</u>   <u>reschedule in</u>_____days weeks months   _____
97124   Exam <u>EMS</u> heat diathermy traction <u>massage</u> ultrasound ice   _____
_____   adjustment: C   D ✓   L ✓   P ✓   extremity   _____
_____   Single   ✓   ✓   ✓   ✓   _____
                          multiple ✓   ____ ____ ____   _____

                                                                                         COMMENTS:

Trt Codes   <u>S:</u>   CERVICAL _____ DORSAL _____ LUMBO-PELVIC ____ _____
_____   <u>O:</u>   spasm C:_____ D:_____L: tender C:____D:_____L:____ _____
_____   <u>A:</u>   improving   unchanged   regressing   temp. relief   _____
_____   <u>P:</u>   reschedule in_____days weeks months   _____
_____   Exam EMS heat diathermy traction massage ultrasound ice   _____
_____   adjustment: C   D   L   P   extremity   _____
                          Single   ____ ____ ____ ____   _____
                          multiple ____ ____ ____ ____   _____

                                                                                         COMMENTS:

Trt Codes   <u>S:</u>   CERVICAL _____ DORSAL _____ LUMBO-PELVIC ____ _____
_____   <u>O:</u>   spasm C:_____ D:_____L: tender C:____D:_____L:____ _____
_____   <u>A:</u>   improving   unchanged   regressing   temp. relief   _____
_____   <u>P:</u>   reschedule in_____days weeks months   _____
_____   Exam EMS heat diathermy traction massage ultrasound ice   _____
_____   adjustment: C   D   L   P   extremity   _____
_____   Single   ____ ____ ____ ____   _____
                          multiple ____ ____ ____ ____   _____

EXAMPLE 7

6/14/94 PTCC: Pain to the right lower back has increased slightly. PT. Used: MH., and Mass. Equip. Used: Treadmill, Isolator and FWs.

6/17/94 PTCC: Right lower back pain has decreased today. PT. Used: MH., and Mass. Equip. Used: Treadmill, FWs and Isolator.

6/20/94 PTCC: Pain into the right lower back has reported to have decreased. PT. Used: Ice, US., MS. and Mass. Equip. Used: Treadmill, Isolator and FWs.

6/21/94 PTCC: Reported some increase in the pain to the right lower back. PT. Used: MH., US., MS. and Mass. Equip. Used: Treadmill, Isolator and FWs.

6/22/94 PTCC: Pain into the right lower back and leg has reported to have decreased slightly. PT. Used: MH., and Mass. Equip. Used: Treadmill, Isolator and FWs.

7/6/94 PTCC: Right lower back and leg painful and tender. PT. Used: MH and Mass.

7/8/94 PTCC: Right lower back and leg pain has increased today. PT. Used: MH. and Mass. Equip. Used: Bike, Treadmill and Isolator.

7/12/94 PTCC; Reported severe pain and spasm in the right lower back and leg PT. Used: Ice and Mass. Equip. Used: Treadmill, Isolator and FWs.

7/13/94 PTCC: Right lower back and leg pain has shown some decrease in intensity today. PT. Used: MH., and Mass. Equip. Used: Treadmill, Isolator and FWs.

7/15/94 PTCC: Right lower back and leg still experiencing pain and spasm. PT. Used: Ice Equip. Used: Treadmill, Isolator and FWs.

7/18/94 PTCC: Pain into the right lower back and leg has shown some decrease today. PT. Used: MH. and US.

7/20/94 PTCC: Slight increase in the,pain to the.right lower back and leg. PT. Used: MH., US. and Mass. Equip. Used: Treadmill, Isolator, and FWs.

7/22/94 PTCC: Small decrease in the pain today to the right lower back and leg. PT. Used: MH. and Mass. Equip. Used: Treadmill, Isolator and FWs.

7/27/94 PTCC: Decreased pain today to the right lower back and leg. PT. Used: Ice and Mass. Equip. Used: Treadmill, Isolator and FWs.

EXAMPLE 8

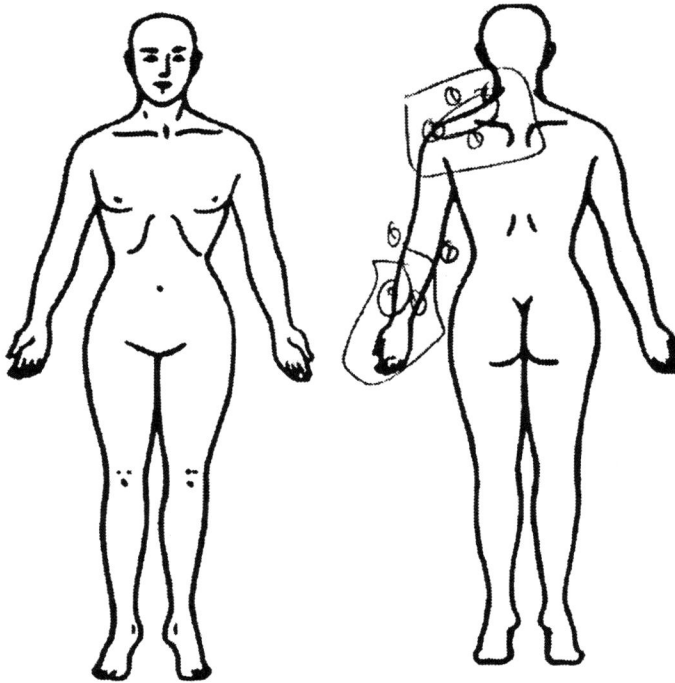

MODALITY	TIME	SETTING	TOLERANCE
6/23/92 ᴴ Us	8 min.	5w cont	H 5:54 us
7/21/92 ᴴ Us	8 min.	5w cont	H 5:45 √ us √
8/17/92 ᴴ Us	8 min	5w cont	H 4:30 us √
9/8/92 ᴴ Us	8 min	5w cont	H 4:55 us √
10/6/92 H,Int Shoulder	10 min	0-150	Int √ H √
10/12/92 H,Int Shoulder	Ice Ant/Hand		Int √ H √
10/26/92 H, Int Shoulder	Ice Ant/Hand	8 min 0-150	H,int √ Ice √
11/9/92 H,Int Shoulder	Ice Ant/Hand	8 min 0-150	H,int √ Ice √
11/30/92 H, Int Shoulder	Ice Ant/Hand	8 min 0-150	H,int √ ice √
12/21/92 H,Int Shoulder	Ice Ant/Hand	8 min 0-150	H,int √ Ice √
1/11/93 H,Int Shoulder	Ice Ant/Hand	8 min 0-150	H,int √ Ice √
2/1/93 H,Int Shoulder	Ice ant/Hand	8 min 0-150	H,int √ Ice √
2/22/93 H,Int Shoulder	Ice Ant/Hand	8 min 0-150	H,int √ Ice √

EXAMPLE 9

Daily Office Notes

NAME:

DATE: 6/2/95

Patient entered the office today complaining of intermittent moderate to severe low back pain and discomfort. Patient stated that she has had one episode of severe low back pain over the last few weeks. Patient stated that she is feeling much better than when the accident first happened. Patient is maintaining a rehabilitation and evaluation schedule of two to three times per week. Patient is progressing satisfactorily. I have released the patient to return to work, but she is being withheld from employment by her work doctor. I feel that it is important to return this patient to work to find out what the effect of her job-related stresses will be on her disc herniation in her low back. Treatment today consisted of a full spine adjustment as indicated by palpation and exercise/rehabilitation. The patient should return two to three times per week.

DATE: 6/6/95

The patient entered the office today for evaluation and rehabilitation. Evaluation of the patient noted subluxations in the lumbar spine. Patient complained of dull aching pain in the low back. Patient is progressing satisfactorily. Treatment today consisted of exercise/rehabilitation and a full spine adjustment as indicated by palpation. Patient should return in two days.

DATE: 6/8/95

Patient entered the office today complaining of low back discomfort. However, the patient has full range of motion and increased function since her work-related injury of 12/17/94. Treatment of the patient today consisted of a full spine adjustment as indicated by palpation and exercise/rehabilitation.

Patient should return two times per week.

EXAMPLE 10

PROGRESS REPORT

PATIENT: PATIENT#

SUPPLEMENTAL REPORT

1. **DATE OF FIRST TREATMENT:** 06-10-95

2. **ORIGINAL DIAGNOSIS:** Lumbar Subluxation 839.2 associated with Lumbar Sprain/Strain 847.2 resulting in a Lumbar Myofascitis 729.1.

3. **UPDATED DIAGNOSIS:** Lumbar Subluxation 839.2 associated with Lumbar Sprain/Strain 847.2 resulting in a Lumbar Myofascitis 729. 1.

4. **DATE OF MOST RECENT EXAM:** 07-05-95

5. **PRESENT SUBJECTIVE COMPLAINTS:** Back pain

6. **PRESENT OBJECTIVE FINDINGS:** Lumbar-limited range of motion with pain, tenderness to palpation, paraspinal muscle tightness, (+) Kemp's Test, (+) Straight leg raiser, (+) Linder's Test, weakness of the quadriceps against resistance, (+) Ely's Test.

7. **INTERIM AGGRAVATIONS OR ACCIDENTS:** Positional stress associated with desk work tends to slow the progress and to exacerbate her condition.

8. **CURRENT STATUS OF PATIENT:** The patient has been reexamined and progress is noted. In accordance with her progress her therapies will be modified to electric muscle stimulation and traction. Home exercises have been modified to include mild abdominal exercises.

9. **PROGNOSIS:** The patient is expected to progress. Due to structural and functional weakness in the lumbar area, she may experience a reoccurrence of symptoms.

10. **THERAPIES:** The goal of electric muscle stimulation and traction is to reduce pain, improve activities of daily living. This is a step towards achieving the long term goals of restoring ROM and ADL, and correcting biomechanical function to as great a degree as possible. The patient will be seen three times weekly and reevaluated in four weeks.

EXAMPLE 11

OBJECTIVE FINDINGS

There were muscle spasm of the:

- ☑ trapezius muscle
- ☑ lower trapezius muscle
- ☐ paraspinal thoracic muscles
- ☐ scalenus anticus muscle
- ☐ levator scapula muscle
- ☐ latissimus dorsi muscle
- ☐ teres minor muscle
- ☑ lumbar erector muscles
- ☐ piriformis muscle
- ☐ paraspinal muscles
- ☐ gluteus maximus muscle
- ☐ gluteus medius muscle
- ☐ psoas muscle
- ☐ deltoid muscle
- ☐ supraspinatous muscle
- ☑ Rhomboideus muscle

POSTURE: Right Left

- ☐ Head Tilt
- ☐ Head Rotation
- ☐ High Shoulder
- ☐ High Ilia

LEG LENGTH   ANTALGIA

Short	R	L	R	L	
			Cervical Spine		
			Thoracic Spine		
			Lumbar Spine		

There was also motion palpation fixation at the level of:

- ☐ C_____ ☐ T_____ ☐ L_____
- ☐ Sacrum_____ ☐ Pelvis_____

☑ This patient is showing decreased range of motion
☐ This patient is showing increased range of motion

ASSESSMENT

The patient

- ☐ is showing some significant improvement
- ☑ is showing very slight improvement; however, noticeable
- ☐ is progressing slowly
- ☐ is progressing poorly
- ☐ suffered an aggravation of the condition

The patient's treatment consisted of:

- ☑ ultrasound
- ☑ mechanical traction
- ☑ myofascial release
- ☐ massage therapy
- ☐ diathermy
- ☑ spinal manipulation
- ☐ microwave
- ☑ + - HVG
- ☐ hot/cold pack
- ☐ flex. distract

PALLIATIVE PLAN

The patient is scheduled to return

- ☐ tomorrow
- ☐ in one week
- ☐ in two weeks
- ☐ as needed
- ☐ in two days
- ☐ twice weekly
- ☐ in ten days
- ☑ three times weekly
- ☐ daily until stabilized
- ☐ in one month

☑ This patient is being followed and evaluated by a neurologist

The patient is being referred out for:

- ☐ an MRI Scan
- ☐ a bone scan
- ☐ blood tests
- ☐ an orthopedic evaluation
- ☐ A CT Scan
- ☐ an EMG
- ☐ a work assessment evaluation
- ☐ a neurological evaluation
- ☐ an EEG
- ☐ a psych. eval.

The patient

- ☐ has been restricted from work
- ☑ is totally disabled at this time
- ☐ has been confined to light duties at work
- ☐ has been permitted to return to work/ light duty only
- ☐ has been permitted to work at normal duties
- ☐ should be at reduced activity
- ☐ is restricted to bed rest
- ☐ is restricted from school
- ☐ is restricted from phys. ed. classes
- ☐ is permitted to return to school

Recommendations

- ☐ Cervical Collar
- ☑ Lumbar Support
- ☑ EMS/ TENS
- ☑ Heat/Ice
- ☐ Orthotics
- ☐ Knee Support
- ☐ Cervical Pillow

PROGNOSIS

- ☑ Guarded
- ☐ Fair
- ☐ Good
- ☐ Excellent

EXAMPLE 12

DATES	SUBJECTIVE	OBJECTIVE	ASSESSMENT	PLANS
7/19/94	Low back pain at arch left foot, right waist pain.	SLR neg to 45 degree, Rt. leg pain when sit to lift	Apparent discopathy L3-4,5.	Treat as prev. DC as needed
7/22/94	Pain lt. thigh, rt. hip, some shoulders, headache	Restriction rt. hip ROM, cervical tense muscles. Lt. foot stiff	Exacerbated yet	Treat: Low volt, spinal manip.
7/29/94	Pain less in neck, rt. hip. No headache but lt. arch	Neck muscles relaxed. Lt. arch stiff, rt. hip	Relief in neck, rt. hip still.	Low volt, manip. Ultrasound
8/17/94	Better this mo. Lt. arch, rt. hip 1/2 ain yet	Neck muscles relaxed. Lt. arch stiff, rt. hip.	Relief in neck, rt. hip still.	Same therapy
8/29/94	Still apin rt. hip, lt. foot	Restr. muscles both.	Not as severe.	Treat as prev.
9/7/94	Same pain areas but better	Restr. less; stiff.	More relief since	Same therapy
12/5/94	Pain lt. neck, foot rt. hip	Stiff lt. neck, foot	ROM less today	Same therapy
2/9/95	Lt. neck, rt. hip-thigh pain	Restr. SLR st. leg.	Under stress 3 da	Same therapy
2/16/95	Still pains all areas	restr. yet, headache	Some improv. but still stressed	Same therapy
4/18/95	Better til yest. pains again hip, foot, neck	Neck stiff, rt. hip, lt. foot restricted	All areas involved not as severe.	Therapy, manip.
5/8/95	Lt. hip pain rt. neck, ankle	Restr. rt. neck, back	Under stress, increased pain.	Therapy, manip.
6/20/95	Pain lt tibial area, low back, rt. hip, lt arch & cervical shiftness=pain.	Restr. all areas & pain in ROM.	Improved after each treat but temporary.	Treat as needed

CRITIQUES

EXAMPLE 1

This is a good example of an initial history. It contains a history about the accident as well as the chief complaint. This also contains information about previous treatment and results.

EXAMPLE 2

This is an example of a reevaluation. The patient's history is taken much like an initial examination. They are asked about their improvement or lack of improvement, job requirements, and activities of daily living. Patients are also asked if they are compliant with home exercises and recommendations.

The reevaluation also includes repeating orthopedic/neurologic tests and updating a clinical impression. The treatment plan is updated to include future treatment frequency, future reevaluations, and work recommendations.

EXAMPLE 3

This example of progress notes contains minimal information. Static listings and a few words are all that is contained in these notes. Remember, the "Gold Standard" for records keeping is a SOAP note format.

EXAMPLE 4

Here is another example of inadequate progress notes. Most of these dates of service contain no subjective history at all. As you can see, it is impossible to tell what the area of complaint is, current subjective and objective findings. There are also no reevaluations found in these notes to help establish the need for continued treatment.

EXAMPLE 5

These are two examples of good SOAP notes, but are more than would be expected under normal circumstances. These are examples of what progress notes look like when transcribed. These examples are actually more that one would typically expect to have for daily progress notes, but are very helpful in following the clinical course of a patient.

EXAMPLE 6

This is an example of progress notes in a "checklist" format. As you can see, the terminology is limited with this style or record keeping. These can be effective if the doctor handwrites notations to make up for the limited vocabulary. If there is no added information, it is difficult to follow a patient's progress is there are twelve consecutive dates where the notation is the same or similar.

EXAMPLE 7

These examples contain only a subjective history and the procedures used on each date of service. As you can see, it is difficult to follow the clinical course with the limited information available. These notes could be enhanced by adding an assessment and treatment plan portion to the notes. This page of notes covers over a month of treatment so there should have been a reexamination. The therapy notes should also contain the location and duration of where the modality is used and there needs to be a key to explain some of the abbreviations.

EXAMPLE 8

This an example of notes for adjunctive modalities. This shows the date, location, time, setting, and modality used. These could be enhanced by providing a key to explain the abbreviations. These could also be written more clearly than they are, but meet the minimum requirements.

EXAMPLE 9

These are examples of daily progress notes. They fulfill the criteria for progress notes. The first record is more complete because it discusses the patient's work status. As you can see, daily progress notes do not have to be lengthy to be effective. This particular patient is in a rehabilitation program and her symptoms have improved so you would not expect significant change from visit to visit.

EXAMPLE 10

This is an example of a reexamination and progress report. I would recommend having more information under "subjective complaints." Explain what activities the patient can now perform that they could not previously perform. This will help show progress or the lack of progress or response to treatment. Also, include how the patient's pain intensity and frequency has improved.

Overall, this is not a bad example of a progress exam. It contains the required elements even though it could be enhanced in some ways.

EXAMPLE 11

This is another example of a "checklist" type of record keeping format. These have a limited vocabulary and terminology and do not always give a clear picture of the patient's clinical picture. It is very hard to follow a patient's progress if you see this type of record keeping on several consecutive dates. Preprinted forms and records should not be constructed solely as a time-saving measure, but they should favor completeness and comprehensives.

EXAMPLE 12

These notes would be sufficient if they were daily progress notes, but what if the first visit was an initial visit? In this case it was. The date of injury was 1992 and the patient presented for treatment on 7/19/94. The prior clinical course is completely unknown. Could you relate this current treatment to injuries sustained in 1992?

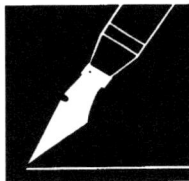

CHAPTER • TWENTY-FIVE

PEER REVIEW SAMPLE CASES

This chapter gives you several case summaries to look at. These are fictitious. As you go through each summary, start to formulate an opinion—Is the diagnosis matching the history and examination? Is there a switch from passive to active? Does the treatment seem appropriate?

There is no exact answer. At the end of each case, we will discuss key points about the case. If you do not see the case as I explain it, don't worry. These are only summaries. Actual cases typically have more documentation and information.

It is time for you to become the examiner!

CASE #1

Date of injury: 8/01/93   Date of review: 9/15/95

Chief Complaint:

Low back pain

History of Occurrence:

The 47-year-old female was injured lifting a box at work. She was bending forward to pick up a box when she felt sudden sharp low back pain.

Past Health History:

History indicates that the patient had lumbar spine surgery in 1990. There was no other past health history presented.

Treatment History:

The patient was initially seen by a Medical Doctor who prescribed medication and a course of physical therapy. The physical therapy consisted of moist heat, ultrasound, ·and exercises. This treatment resulted in no clinical change. The patient also had trials of several medications with no significant improvement. The medical treatment lasted from the date of injury until 2/15/94.

She presented for chiropractic treatment on 2/21/94. She complained of constant low back pain that radiated down the left leg. Examination revealed decreased lumbar ROM, positive SLR, positive Braggard's, and positive WLR. There were no reflex, sensory, or motor abnormalities in the lower extremities.

A lumbar MRI dated 4/92 showed narrowing at L4/5 and post-surgical changes at this same level.

Diagnosis:

Acute lumbar spine pain complicated by degenerative changes and post-surgical changes.

Treatment:

Myofascial release, adjustments, and interferential.

The patient was treated 47 times through 11/21/94 when she reached MMI and was placed on a PRN basis. She was treated 12 times from 11/21/94-10/10/95. The current treatment is the result of the patient's need to present for symptomatic exacerbations only. The patient continues to work at her occupation at least 40 hours per week.

Question:

Is the current PRN treatment reasonable and necessary in relation to injuries received on 8/1/93?

This case could be a candidate for supportive care. Do you remember the criteria for supportive care? If not, you can review the criteria for supportive care in Chapter 2. With the history of surgery and post-surgical changes this patient should be afforded the opportunity for supportive care. The treatment of 12 times in almost 11 months would be considered reasonable. Supportive care is typically rendered at the frequency of one to two times per month.

Is the use of the word "acute" in the diagnosis appropriate? NO. The word acute would only be appropriate for the first 6-8 weeks following the injury.

CASE #2

History of Occurrence:

The 27-year-old patient was stopped at a red light when he was struck from behind by another car. He said he was not wearing his seatbelt at the time of the accident and struck his head on the windshield. He did not require any emergency treatment the day of the accident.

Past Medical History:

Unremarkable. He works as a "cutter" in the clothing factory.

Treatment History:

He was treated the following day in the emergency room. He was x-rayed and examined. He complained of neck pain. The x-rays of the neck were unremarkable. He was prescribed a muscle relaxer and instructed to go to the rehabilitation clinic the next day. He was diagnosed with a myoligamentous sprain and prescribed a course of physical therapy consisting of moist heat and exercises. He was seen 6 times at the physical therapy department and released. This treatment lasted three weeks.

One week later he presented to the office of Harvey Lillard, D.C. No exam findings, treatment plan, diagnosis, or reexams were found. Treatment consisted of hot packs, spinal adjustments, and intersegmental traction. He was seen 30 times over the course of 12 weeks.

Four weeks after starting treatment with Dr. Lillard, he was examined by Dr. Spok (also a D.C.). Dr. Spok took more x-rays that were said to show an "unstable cervical situation." (There were no flexion/extension studies.) There were no examination findings, diagnosis, or treatment plan from Dr. Spok provided for review.

The patient treated with both DCs for six months. He apparently did not like to wait so he would go to the doctor who was not as busy. Currently, he is adjusted from 2 times a week to one time every 3-4 weeks.

Question:

Comment on the reasonableness and necessity of past, present and future care.

There was a clinical course from the time of injury to when he presented for chiropractic treatment. In other words, there was no significant gaps between the types of treatment. Neither doctor provided a clinical examination, diagnosis, treatment, plan, or reexaminations. Doctors must first establish the need for treatment by performing the appropriate history, examination, and formulating a treatment plan.

Since there was a mechanism of injury that would contribute to a musculoskeletal diagnosis, it may be reasonable to allow for a trial of chiropractic care. The patient was treating with two doctors at once with no communication between the doctors. The second doctor should have taken an adequate history and known about the first course of chiropractic treatment. What would you do? I am usually inclined to go with the treatment of the first doctor as long as it is medically necessary. The second chiropractor should have tried to communicate with the first doctor. Concurrent treatment may be reasonable as long as both chiropractors are in communication.

Were the repeat x-rays by both chiropractors medically necessary? There was insufficient documentation to justify the repeat exposure of the x-rays. The hospital x-rays should have been viewed to determine whether additional studies were indicated.

CASE #3

Date of Injury: 11/17/93   Date of Review: 6/1/95

History of Occurrence:

The patient was the belted driver of a car that was stopped and struck from behind by another auto. She was taken to the ER by ambulance where she was x-rayed and treated. The x-rays did not reveal a fracture or dislocation and the patient was released the same day.

Past Health History:

The patient was previously diagnosed with stenosis of the abdominal aorta. She smokes two packs of cigarettes per day. She has a chronic cough and COPD. She is also taking several medications.

Treatment History:

She presented for treatment with Dr. Still who is a D.O. He diagnosed "cervical sprain/strain with multiple osteopathic lesions, and thoracic and lumbar sprain/strain." The treatment consisted of medications and osteopathic manipulation. She was treated four times over four weeks and released to go back to work.

A course of physical therapy consisting of hot packs, ultrasound, and flexibility exercises was initiated on 1/27/94. These records were not provided for this peer review.

The patient underwent an MRI on 12/29/93. This study revealed minimal central disc bulging at L3-4 and C5-6.

A neurology report indicated that there was the presence of cervical and lumbar spine radiculopathies on electrodiagnostic tests.

On 11/22/93 the patient presented for chiropractic care. There were no examination, progress notes, or treatment plan provided for review. There were also no reexaminations.

The diagnosis was chronic ligament sprain with cervical subluxation. Treatment was recommended at three times a week for six months, however, treatment was rendered at a frequency of 4 to 6 times per month.

A progress report to the insurance carrier indicates that the doctor gave her a 10% permanent impairment on 6/22/94. He continued to treat on a regular basis. Bills showed services to be office visits and temperature measurement in the form of a 3R thermograph on each date of service.

Questions:

1. Does the medical documentation support the appropriateness of care rendered?

2. Does the information support the need for a permanent impairment rating?

3. Is the use of the decade 3-R thermograph medically necessary?

Due to the patient's clinical course and prior history, a trial of chiropractic care would be appropriate. However, to evaluate the efficacy of treatment and establish the need for continued treatment, reexaminations need to be performed. Since no examinations were performed, the treatment would not have been justified past 60-90 days. The patient also has complicating factors that would have prolonged recovery.

The permanent impairment rating would not be substantiated. The attending doctor gave the patient a permanent impairment then continued to treat on a regular basis. A permanent impairment is only given when a patient has reached a static point after which they would not see significant improvement. If the impairment is "permanent" no regular treatment would be needed. In this case, the impairment rating would not be justified because the doctor continued to treat on a scheduled basis in an attempt to achieve clinical gains.

The use of the decade 3-R thermography is not considered medically necessary. This is used preparatory to the adjustment and would be considered part of the adjustment or office visit. It would not be considered medically necessary because it does not contribute to the differential diagnosis, prognosis, or therapeutic plan.

CASE #4

Date of injury: 9/30/94   Date of review: 4/20/96

History of occurrence:

The patient was moving a chair at work when she leaned back onto her heel and felt a sudden pulling sensation in her right hip and pain down the outside of her right leg to her heel.

Past Medical History:

The patient was diagnosed with carpal tunnel syndrome in 1990. She underwent carpal tunnel syndrome release in her right hand in 1991. She continues to have pain and numbness in both hands.

Treatment history:

The patient initially saw an orthopod who ordered an MRI that showed sacralization of L5. Physical therapy was ordered that consisted of ultrasound, moist heat, and exercises for four weeks. This resulted in no significant improvement.

The patient then saw a D.C. for 6 weeks. Spinal adjustments and ultrasound offered temporary relief. She was also seen by a neurologist who diagnosed bursitis and treated the patient with cortisone injections.

She presented to the chiropractor under review on 8/3/95. Initial exam findings consisted of: "pulling" on cervical and lumbar range of motion; positive Kemp's on right; positive Tinel's bilaterally; +2/4 upper extremity reflexes.(these were the only tests done).

A diagnostic ultrasound was ordered to "determine the level of inflammation." Upper and lower extremity NCVs were ordered to "asses radiculopathies vs. CTS." The upper extremity NCV showed left carpal tunnel syndrome. A lower extremity EMG/NCV was ordered and found to be unremarkable. Lumbar spine x-rays showed sacralization of L5.

Diagnosis:

"Grade 2 sprain/strain of the lumbar spine with associated HNP and suspected radiculopathy." "Failed carpal tunnel syndrome surgery."

Treatment:

Intersegmental traction, flexion distraction, spinal adjustments, extremity adjustments, myofascial release, and ultrasound. There were 58 dates of service from 8/3/95 to 3/28/96 which is the last date of service provided for review. There was a gap in treatment from 12/6/95-1/6/96. Treatment notes indicate that the patient was being treated for right and left carpal tunnel syndrome, neck and upper back pain, low back pain, and suspected hypothyroidism. Lumbar spine range of motion was redone on 9/12/95 and 1/13/96. Throughout the first 30 visits, the low back complaint was mentioned only five times.

Questions:

1. Can the diagnosis be supported by the examination findings?

2. Comment on the medical necessity of the ancillary diagnostic tests?

3. Comment on the reasonableness and necessity of care in relation to injuries sustained on 9/30/94.

The MRI and examination did not reveal any signs of disc involvement, so this part of the diagnosis would not be supported. The examination shows continued signs of carpal tunnel syndrome so the "failed carpal tunnel syndrome" is reasonable, but is this part of the diagnosis related to the work related injury?

The rationale for the diagnostic ultrasound is not appropriate based on the information available. The clinical examination should have been sufficient to locate the level of involvement. Does the diagnostic ultrasound contribute to the differential diagnosis, prognosis, or therapeutic plan?

The upper and lower extremity NCV/EMGs would not be medically necessary and reasonable. The appropriate clinical examination was not performed prior to ordering these tests. (This is a very common mistake.) Using ancillary diagnostic tests without first establishing the need is not appropriate. A complete exam would include orthopedic tests and motor, reflex, and sensory examination of the extremities. Also, the upper extremity testings would not relate to this date of injury.

A large portion of care in this case would not be reasonable. The injuries that were sustained on the date of injury under review was to the low back only. Most of the dates of service did not even mention the low back but were directed to the cervical spine and wrists. This is an example of a patient with multiple problems.

The treating doctor must be aware of who is responsible for each particular injury when third party issues are involved.

Each case must be looked at carefully!

CASE #5

Date of review: 4/19/96

History of occurrence:

The patient is a 19-year-old female who was injured in an automobile accident on 1/23/95. She was the unbelted back seat passenger of an automobile that could not get stopped and rear-ended another car on a major highway. Immediately she was taken by ambulance to the emergency room were she was x-rayed and examined. Her complaints were of neck and back pain. The x-rays were unremarkable. Treatment consisted of a cervical collar, medication, and warm compresses 4 times a day.

Treatment History:

On 12/6/95, the patient presented for chiropractic treatment with complaints of neck pain, back pain, and headaches. The patient is a student. She indicates using Advil for the pain and has not sought care since being treated in the emergency room. Examination revealed negative cervical compression and distraction. Tenderness was noted in the cervical spine musculature.

Diagnosis:

"The effects of acute traumatic acceleration/deceleration injury including myospasm, myofascitis, segmental dysfunction, and tension headaches as a direct result."

Treatment:

Treatment consisted of spinal adjustments, massage, and home stretches. Treatment was recommended at the frequency of two times per week for 24 weeks. Progress notes show 6 dates of service from 12/6/95 through 1/5/96. There was a gap in treatment from 1/5/96 through 3/29/96.

Question:

Does all of the care appear to be causally related?

You must look carefully at the dates in this case. The patient was treated in a car accident on 1/23/95. She was treated on that date. She did not present for care until 12/6/95 which is over ten months later. Causality would be difficult to establish. The patient is a student carrying a bookbag over her shoulders, studying with her head flexed for long periods of time, and involved in athletics. These would all contribute to a cervical spine complaint and make the examiner question if the present complaints were causally related to the MVA.

CASE #6

Date of injury: 5/23/90   Date of review: 1/15/96

History of Occurrence:

The patient was working on an earth mover when he fell onto the ground landing on his mid back. The 50-year-old male was taken immediately to the emergency room where he was x-rayed and diagnosed with compression fractures of the mid back.

Treatment History:

The patient treated with an orthopod from the date of the injury to 7/29/91 when he presented for chiropractic treatment. His chief complaint was constant mid back pain. He had been treated medically with several courses of physical therapy and medications but continued to have constant pain.

Plain film x-rays dated 5/23/90 and 7/29/91 show compression fractures and healed compression fractures, respectively, at T6 and T11.

The chiropractic treatment consisted of spinal adjustments and TENS. The diagnosis was "complications of two crushed backbones." Progress notes indicate that the patient responds to chiropractic care. Treatment withdrawal results in deterioration of the patient. The progress notes show 115 dates of service from 12/20/95. Current treatment frequency is 1 to 2 times per month on a PRN basis.

Questions:

1. Is the current treatment reasonable and necessary for injuries sustained on 5/23/90? (Remember the criteria for supportive care)

The diagnosis is certainly descriptive. I feel that the patient has met the criteria for supportive care. There are documented complaints that respond to chiropractic care. Treatment is rendered on a PRN basis in response to symptomatic exacerbations. Alternative treatments had been attempted but had previously been unsuccessful and there had been trial of treatment withdrawal.

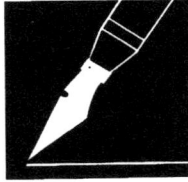

CHAPTER TWENTY-SIX

SAMPLE PEER REVIEW REPORTS

These are examples of peer review reports. They are to assist the reviewer in understanding the review format and how a report is written. They are not designed to be used as a "cookbook" approach to writing a report. Each case is different and this should be reflected in the writing of the report. The names are fictional and do not represent anyone in particular.

December 9, 1996

Claimant: Tom Jones
SS#: 888-66-5555
D/I: 2/14/96
Review#: 40885

To Whom It May Concern,

I have reviewed the medical records in the above-mentioned case for the purpose of a retrospective review.

The following information is based solely upon submitted records which are listed below, absent the opportunity to personally examine the patient.

RECORDS REVIEWED:
- UR assignment
- UR request
- Roger Doger, D.C.:
  - Medical report forms
  - History and Diagnosis
  - Progress notes 5/30/96–11/8/96
- McDonald Chiropractic:
  - Confidential patient information 2/17/96
  - Past health history
  - Accident report 2/17/96
  - Neck disability index

Page 2
Tom Jones

- Examinations 2/16/96, 5/2/96
- Progress notes 2/16/96–5/2/96

CASE REVIEW:

The claimant, Tom Jones, was reported to have sustained injuries in a work related accident on 2/14/96. He was the belted driver of a vehicle that lost control on the ice traveling at approximately 25 miles an hour. He was driving to a bankruptcy hearing at the time of the accident.

On 2/17/96 he presented to the office of McDonald Chiropractic for examination and treatment. Complaints include neck, mid-back and low-back pain. Examination revealed: decreased cervical spine range of motion with pain, positive Foraminal Compression and Shoulder Depressor tests, decreased sensation in the C7,8 dermatomes on the right, decreased lumbar spine range of motion, positive Kemp's, positive Laseque's, positive Valsalva's, positive Soto Hall, and positive Milgram's.

The initial diagnosis included: cervical sprain/strain, cervicalgia, subluxations, pain in the thoracic spine, thoracic sprain/strain, and lumbalgia. The initial treatment was recommended at the frequency of three times a week for four weeks. Treatment consisted of spinal adjustments, electrical muscle stimulation, diathermy, and hot packs.

Progress notes show 22 dates of service from 2/16/96 through 5/2/96. The patient was discharged on 5/2/96 due to not following recommended treatment.

On 5/30/96 the claimant presented to the office of Roger Doger, D.C. for examination and treatment. A medical report dated 6/6/96 indicates a diagnosis of thoracic and cervical sprain, cervical whiplash syndrome, and previous lumbar radiculopathy. Treatment consisted of adjustments, interferential, and hot packs.

The progress notes show 16 dates of service from 5/30/96 through 11/8/96. There were no complete initial examination findings provided for review. There were gaps in treatment from 6/4-6/27, 7/12-8/29, and 10/3-10/25. He was apparently having problems keeping the treatment schedule.

PHONE CONSULTATION:

There was no phone consultation requested.

CLINICAL OPINION:

I have been asked to address the reasonableness and necessity of care provided to Tom Jones by Roger Doger, D.C. from 9/10/96 and ongoing. Based upon the submitted records, the reasonableness and necessity of care has been established in part for the following reasons:

- The claimant was injured in an auto accident during the course of his employment. He was diagnosed as suffering cervical and thoracic sprains as well as aggravating a low back condition. He had undergone a course of chiropractic care from McDonald Chiropractic but was discharged due to noncompliance.
- Mr. Jones consulted Roger Doger, D.C. for treatment. The treatment was again erratic due to noncompliance. I feel that treatment rendered through and including 10/3/96 would appear reasonable. At this time, the treatment again

Page 3
Tom Jones

became sporadic. Treatment on an irregular basis such as this after this period of time would not result in a clinical progression. I do not feel that treatment beyond 10/3/96 would be reasonable for injuries sustained on 2/14/96.

CLOSURE:

The opinions rendered in this case are those of the reviewer. This review has been conducted without medical examination of the individual reviewed. This is based on documents provided to us by the provider with the assumption that the diagnosis is true and correct. This report is a clinical assessment and opinion conducted with the information available. It does not constitute per se recommendations for specific claims to be made or enforced.

Sincerely,

Hack-U-Up, D.C.

December 26, 1996

Claimant: Sally Smith
Review#: 6683-WIN
D/I: 4/21/96
DOB: 6/10/84
CL#: 4444444DC

To Whom It May Concern,

I have reviewed the medical records in the above-mentioned case for the purpose of a retrospective review.

The following information is based solely upon submitted records which are listed below, absent the opportunity to personally examine the patient.

RECORDS REVIEWED:

- Authorization and assignment of benefits
- Mable Palmer DC
  - Letter to Ins. Co. 12/10/96
  - History and Examination page
  - Case history, undated
  - Initial report 5/6/96
  - "Updated subjective complaints" 7/31/96, 9/18/96
  - Progress Report 7/31/96
  - Date of service page
  - Progress notes 5/8/96–12/2/96

CASE REVIEW:

Sally Smith was involved in an automobile accident on 4/21/96. She was the belted right rear passenger of an automobile that was stopped at a red light and struck from behind. The application for benefits indicates the vehicle she was riding in was a van, but a letter dated 12/10/96 from Palmer Chiropractic indicates the vehicle was a Lumina. There was no indication of the extent of the damage or if any emergency treatment was received.

Miss Smith presented to the office of Dr. Mable Palmer for examination and treatment on 5/6/96. An undated case history indicates a complaint of "stiffness" for three days' duration. Initial examination findings consisted of decreased cervical spine range of motion. It is unclear whether any other examinations were performed. The initial diagnosis was "traumatic cephalgia and hyperflexion/hyperextension injury." There was no x-ray report supplied for review. A letter dated 12/10/96 to Allstate indicates that cervical spine x-rays revealed a hypolordotic cervical spine and foraminal encroachment from C5-T1.

The initial report dated 5/6/96 indicates treatment utilized includes: manipulation, traction, ultrasound, "brace," heat, cold, EMS, cervical pillow and exercises. A progress report dated 7/31/96 indicates that a rehabilitation exercise program for strengthening was to be done at the frequency of 2 to 3 times a week for 4 weeks.

Progress notes show 50 dates of service from 5/8/96 to 12/2/96. The progress notes are in a semi-coded format with no key provided for review. There are

Page 2
Sally Smith

several dates where there was no subjective notation in the medical file. It is also unknown from whom the history was obtained. The case history is written in a child's handwriting but signed by the mother. The updated subjective complaints dated 7/31/96 indicating the complaints "didn't change a lot" is also in a child's handwriting.

PHONE CONSULTATION WITH THE ATTENDING DOCTOR:

On 12/17/96 I had the opportunity to speak with Dr. Palmer regarding her treatment of Sally Smith. Dr. Palmer indicated that she will release Miss Smith tomorrow if she remains improved. Dr. Palmer said that the response to treatment was slower than expected. According to Dr. Palmer, Miss Smith experienced neck pain and headaches as result of the accident. Dr. Palmer indicated that her care included a home strengthening protocol for 4 weeks.

CLINICAL OPINION:

I have been asked to address the reasonableness and necessity of care provided to Sally Smith by Mable Palmer, D.C. Specifically, I have been asked if the treatment is medically necessary, reasonable, and appropriate as a result of injuries sustained on 4/21/96.

I do agree with the application of chiropractic care to a degree in the management of this case. Miss Smith was first examined on 5/6/96 for complaints that were attributed to the automobile accident. She was treated 8 to 9 times a month in May, June, and July and 6 times in August. The examination of 7/31/96 only contained a range of motion assessment.

Treatment through 8/21/96 would have been sufficient in treating this child. Due to the patient's age, a reasonable course of treatment would include spinal adjustments and no more than one adjunctive modality per date of service at of frequency of one time per week.

The treatment included a four-week strengthening home exercise program starting at the end of July. It would be reasonable to monitor the child on a weekly basis while undergoing this program. However, it is unclear why passive care was again started at the end of this active care phase. Active care is typically the end point of care unless a symptomatic exacerbation occurs. There was no documentation in the medical file to support the continued application of passive modalities after the active phase of care.

There was also no objective means for quantifying whether the strength gains that were desired were in fact attained. There was also a gap in treatment from 8/21/96 through 9/3/96 during which no treatment was received.

The treatment plan that was rendered to this child would have been more consistent with treating an adult and not an eleven year old. Certain modalities and exercises would be contraindicated when treating a child of this age because of the considerations of the growing epiphysis. Based upon the patient's own self-evaluation on 7/31/96, it is unclear if the treatment rendered to this point did, in fact, help. It would not be reasonable to continue treatment with no subjective or objective findings to substantiate continued treatment. The minimally informative

Page 3
Sally Smith

nature of the progress notes doe not accurately reflect the clinical status of the child.

CLOSURE:

The opinions rendered in this case are the opinions of the reviewer. This review has been conducted without a medical examination of the individual reviewed. This is based on documents provided to us by the provider with the assumption that the diagnosis is true and correct. This report is a clinical assessment and opinion conducted with the information available. It does not constitute per se recommendation for specific claims to be made or enforced.

Sincerely,

Dee Nye, D.C.

8/10/95

Hatchet Man Reviews, Inc.

1313 Luck Lane

Yourtown, PA 11111

RE: Gary Smith

D/I: 2/26/93

To Whom It May Concern,

I have reviewed the medical records in the above-mentioned case for the purpose of a retrospective review.

The following information is based solely upon submitted records which are listed below, absent the opportunity to personally examine the patient.

RECORDS REVIEWED:

- 4 page report dated 12/20/93
- 6 pages of billing audits showing 41 dates of service from 3/4/93 through 9/30/93.

CASE REVIEW:

The patient, Gary Smith, was reported to have sustained injuries in a car accident on 2/26/93. He was the passenger in a car that was stopped and struck from behind by a taxicab. He was not wearing his seatbelt.

Immediately following the accident, he was taken to Hahnemann Hospital where his neck was x-rayed and he was released.

On 3/4/93, he presented to the office of Dr. Fisher for examination and treatment. He had decreased cervical and lumbar ranges of motion. Foraminal Compression and Laseque's tests were positive. Lumbar spine x-rays were negative for fracture of dislocation. Treatment has consisted of passive modalities and spinal adjustments.

The initial diagnosis was "post traumatic cervical and lumbar spine instability" and "grade two cervical and thoracolumbar myoligamentous sprain." He was discharged from care on 9/30/93 with no residuals. Records show 41 dates of service form 3/4/93 through 9/30/93.

CLINICAL OPINION:

I have been asked to address the seriousness of the injury, extent of the injury and whether a permanent injury has resulted.

1. The injuries that were sustained were not significant enough to be considered a "serious impairment of a bodily function." The diagnosis of cervical and lumbar spine instability is not substantiated by valid objective clinical findings.

2. Mr. Smith would not have a permanent impairment based on the AMA Guides to the Evaluation of Permanent Impairment. He was released with no residuals and this was well-documented in the clinical records. A notation in the medical file states "his instabilities have responded to treatment and normal spinal biomechanics have returned."

Thank you for allowing me to participate in this case.

Sincerely,

Dr. Lillard

November 24, 1995

RE: Lisa Smith
SS: 111-22-3333
D/I: 9/2/93
Review#: 88888

Dear Sir/Madam:

In response to your request, I have provided a reconsideration review pertaining to the patient, Lisa Smith. The report contains my assessment of chiropractic care documented for this individual. No physical examination of the patient has been requested. The opinions expressed in this report solely reflect my assessment of the available records.

MEDICAL DOCUMENTS REVIEWED:
- Request for review
- Correspondence, My Town Chiro. Center
- Daily office notes, 9/9/93 through 9/30/95
- Patient history 9/2/93
- Diagnostic reports, 1/29/94, 7/11/95
- Employer's report of occupational injury
- Work/Comp questionnaire 9/ 16/93
- Medical reports and initial report

CASE REVIEW:

The patent, Lisa Smith, reportedly sustained injuries in a work-related accident on 9/2/93. The patient reported injury while bending under a desk to pick up garbage. The patient first sought chiropractic treatment on 9/9/93. The attending chiropractor diagnosed the patient with post-traumatic chronic dorsal radiculopathy, post-traumatic chronic cervical sprain/strain, post-traumatic chronic lumbosacral iliac sprain/strain. The chiropractic treatment program had consisted of a physical examination, moist heat packs, massage therapy, manual traction, electrical stimulation, and spinal manipulation. The course of chiropractic care documented in this file had consisted of 39 visits from 9/9/93 to 2/5/94. There was an absence in chiropractic treatment until the patient re-presented on 7/13/95.

The patient received an additional 9 visits through 9/30/95.

In addition to chiropractic care, the patient underwent several different ancillary diagnostic procedures including x-rays and an MRI scan. X-rays taken in September of 1993 were unremarkable. The MRI performed on 1/28/94 demonstrated a normal appearance of the thoracic spine.

There is no significant explanation for the lapse in treatment from February 1994 until the patient presented for care in July 1995. The history of the patient's clinical status in the interim is not described. The patient's complaint include mid back pain and moderate to severe low back pain.

Page 2
Lisa Smith

DISCUSSION WITH THE ATTENDING CHIROPRACTOR:

On 11/21/95, I had the opportunity to speak with the attending chiropractor concerning Ms. Smith. Dr. X stated he was currently seeing Ms. Smith on an as-needed basis. Dr. X noted complications of obesity and diabetes mellitus. This doctor recommended future care on an as needed basis.

CONCLUSIONS AND RECOMMENDATIONS:

I have received a request for my opinion regarding the reasonableness and necessity of all chiropractic treatment from 7/27/95 and into the future.

In assessing the available information, it is my opinion that the reasonableness and necessity of chiropractic services has not been established from 7/27/95 and after. The patient had sustained a sprain/strain injury in September of 1993. The patient had discontinued trials of treatment management in 2/94 for this acute injury. The patient did not present for care in the management of this condition until 7/13/95. This pattern of presentation is not consistent with management for a sprain/strain injury. Objective findings are limited in assessing the etiology of the radicular syndrome reported. Inconsistency in the management of this condition does not support expectations of further clinical progression with the utilization of conservative treatment measures.

In essence, the records provided have not substantiated the reasonableness and necessity of continued chiropractic treatment management from 7/27/95 and into the future.

Thank you for requesting this assessment.

Sincerely,

Dr. Dee Nye

October 23, 1995

RE: Helen Smith

SS#: 000-11-2222

D/I: 5/15/92

To Whom It May Concern,

I have received the medical documentation on the above-referenced patient, Helen Smith, to perform a review of records. Specifically, I was asked to comment upon the reasonableness and necessity of chiropractic treatment provided Helen Smith by Hillary Rodman, D.C. from 7/17/95 and ongoing.

The following clinical opinions are based solely upon submitted records which are listed below, absent the opportunity to personally examine the patient. These opinions are based upon clinical experience, common standards of medical necessity, and the assumption that the information provided in these records is correct. The clinical opinions provided do not constitute a recommendation for a specific claim or administrative function to be made of enforced. Final benefit determinations are the sole responsibility of the insurance carrier.

DOCUMENTATION REVIEWED:

- Peer review request
- Utilization review assignment
- Reconsideration request
- Correspondence, Hillary Rodman, D.C., 10/3/95, 11/4/94
- Laboratory report, 6/16/95
- Nerve Conduction Velocity, 9/10/92
- Correspondence, Paul Slice, M.D., 7/28/94, 6/19/94
- MRI Report, 6/17/92
- Case history, 6/8/92
- Treatment notes, 6/8/92 through 9/6/95

SUMMARY OF RECORDS REVIEWED:

According to the records submitted, Mrs. Smith presented to the office of Hillary Rodman, D.C. on 6/8/92 with complaints of pain in the wrists and hands accompanied by numbness, tingling, loss of strength, frequent headaches, sweats, stiffness and pain in the neck radiating to the mid scapular area, cold hands, chest pains, and other manifestations of circulatory compromise. It was noted that the patient first noted these symptoms in May of 1992 while working at Bad Meats, Inc. She initially was seen by the company doctor who prescribed physical therapy and released Mrs. Smith to return to work.

Initial examination by Dr. Rodman resulted in diagnostic impression of cervicalgia, lower cervical radiculitis, upper extremity paresthesia, and carpal tunnel syndrome. There were 351 dates submitted for review from 6/8/92 through 9/6/95. During the period of time in question, there were 23 dates of service from 7/17/95 through 9/6/95. Treatment consisted of spinal adjustments and electrical stimulation. The patient was advised to return for treatment on a three-times-a-week basis.

Page 2
Helen Smith

In addition to the chiropractic care, the patient was also evaluated and/or treated by the following practitioners:

1. Paul Slice, M.D. He recommended anti-inflammatory agents and muscle relaxers.

2. Feel Good, M.D. Dr. Good diagnosed thoracic outlet syndrome and recommended neck exercises and medication.

The following diagnostic tests results were submitted for review:

1. Transcranial Doppler Study, 6/14/95 that was normal.

2. NCV, 9/10/92. This revealed possible left thoracic outlet syndrome but was otherwise normal.

3. Cervical spine MRI, 6/17/92. This was reported to be negative.

CLINICAL OPINION:

I have been asked to comment upon the reasonableness and necessity of chiropractic treatment provided to Helen Smith by Hillary Rodman, D.C. from 7/17/95 and ongoing.

In assessing the records provided, it is my opinion that reasonableness and necessity of chiropractic treatment from 7/17/95 and ongoing has not been established for the following reasons:

1. Review of records revealed the continuous unaltered application of passive therapy consisting of spinal adjustments and electrical stimulation at a constant frequency of three times a week throughout the entire course of treatment form 6/8/92 through 9/6/95. Submitted treatment notes documented persistent subjective complaints and only contained static listings. Although there was no indication of clinical improvement in the patient's condition, the patient continued to treat at a frequency of three visits per week. Where a significant reduction in treatment frequency is not noted, as in this particular case, it is reasonable to conclude that the patient's response to treatment was not optimal and, therefore, either alteration in the treatment protocol or discontinuation of treatment would be indicated.

2. Submitted documentation did not include periodic reexamination findings. There were no clear objective measures that would support the need for ongoing passive chiropractic treatment at the constant frequency of three visits per week.

Sincerely,

Cut-U-Off DC

February 28, 1996

RE: John Jones
SS#:999-88-7777
D/I: 6/9/94
Review#: 99222

To Whom It May Concern,

I have received the medical documentation on the above-referenced patient, John Jones, to perform a review of records. Specifically, I was asked to comment upon the reasonableness and necessity of chiropractic treatment provided John Jones by Joe Toggle, D.C. from 8/10/95 and ongoing.

The following clinical opinions are based solely upon submitted records which are listed below, absent the opportunity to personally examine the patient. These opinions are based upon clinical experience, common standards of medical necessity, and the assumption that the information provided in these records is correct. The clinical opinions provided do not constitute a recommendation for a specific claim or administrative function to be made of enforced. Final benefit determinations are the sole responsibility of the insurance carrier.

DOCUMENTATION REVIEWED:

- Peer review request, 2/22/96
- Request for reconsideration
- Progress reports, Joe Toggle, D.C.
- Examination findings, 6/13/94, 2/28/95, 4/10/95
- Treatment notes 6/13/94-11/2/95
- Radiology reports, 6/9/94, 4/27/95
- MRI report, 4/27/95
- Report Bill Smith, M.D., 4/19/95
- Progress notes, St. John's Health Center

SUMMARY OF RECORDS REVIEWED:

According to the submitted records, John Jones, a 36-year-old male, presented into the office of Joe Toggle, D.C. for examination and treatment of injuries reportedly sustained in an accident on 6/9/94. It was reported that Mr. Jones was lifting up a shield on a machine when he flipped over landing on a catwalk. He was treated and released from St. John's Health Center. X-rays of the pelvis and lumbosacral spines were negative. The diagnosis from St. John's was "acute contusion of the back."

On 6/13/94 Mr. Jones presented to Dr. Toggle with complaints of low back pain, pain down the left leg to the heel, left leg numbness, upper back stiffness, and left sided neck pain. Initial diagnosis was lumbar sprain/strain.

Mr. Jones had a previous injury in 1990. He underwent surgery for a herniated lumbar disc. Surgery resulted in relief of pain and Mr. Jones was able to return to work.

Page 2
John Jones

Submitted for review was record of 3 dates of chiropractic treatment from 6/13/94 through 6/16/94, no record of care from 6/17/94 through 11/16/94, resumption of treatment on 11/17/94 through 11/21/94 for 2 visits and no care again from 11/22/94 through 2/23/95. Records indicate Mr. Jones returned for care on 2/24/95 and received 8 treatments including 4/10/95. There was again no records from 4/11/95 through 8/9/95. Mr. Jones subsequently was treated on 3 occasions from 8/10/95 to and including 11/2/95. There was no record of treatment subsequent to 11/2/95. Treatment included spinal adjustments, traction, and interferential therapy.

Bill Smith, M.D. was consulted on 4/19/95 regarding the recurrence of left sciatica. Dr. Smith's impression included possible recurrent disc herniation. Mr. Smith recommended an MRI and updated lumbar spine x-rays. The MRI showed no evidence of recurrent disc herniation and narrowing at L5/S1. He recommended low back exercises.

TELEPHONE CONVERSATION WITH THE ATTENDING DOCTOR:

On 2/28/96 I had the opportunity to speak with Dr. Toggle regarding the current clinical status of Mr. Jones. Dr. Toggle reported the patient received a permanent injury which necessitates present and future chiropractic treatment. Treatment consists of manipulation, ice, traction, interferential, and home exercises. Dr. Toggle indicated that the patient is a construction worker and experiences occasional periodic exacerbations of his condition.

CLINICAL OPINION:

I have been asked to address the reasonableness and necessity of care from 8/10/95 and ongoing. In assessing the records provided, it is my opinion, that the reasonableness and necessity of chiropractic care rendered on an as-needed basis as a pain management program from 8/10/95 and ongoing has been established. The level of chiropractic treatment provided by the attending chiropractor appears to fall within general treatment expectations of a supportive care program designed to address the sequel which has arisen from the chronic condition described in this case.

As to the issue of continuing chiropractic care, it is my opinion that the patient's chronic condition warrants a pain management program reflective of chiropractic care rendered on an as-needed basis. Of course, as part of supportive phase of care a limited frequency of presentation would be anticipated. One would not expect the frequency of supportive care not to exceed 1 to 2 visits per month for the management of this condition. In order for an as-needed treatment to be appropriate it should not be prescheduled and should be provided solely in response to a documented date of exacerbation.

Sincerely,

A. Proved, D.C.

April 1, 1997

RE: Jill Jack
CO#: 8888
DOA: 6/1/96

I have reviewed the medical records provided on the above-mentioned claimant. The following opinion is based solely upon submitted records which are listed below, absent the opportunity to personally examine the patient.

RECORDS REVIEWED:
- Authorization
- Peer review report, Dee Nye, D.C., 12/1/96
- Cervical and Lumbar X-ray reports
- Cervical and Lumbar MRI reports
- EMG/NCV
- B. J. Adio, D.C.
  - Progress notes 6/21/96–10/17/96
  - HCFA Billings
  - Oswestry and Neck Disability Index
  - Letters to Ins. Co.
- Sam Mixer, D.C.
  - History and Examination 11/5/96
  - Progress notes 6/21/96–10/17/96
  - Reexamination 12/6/96
  - HCFA Billings

CASE REVIEW:

Jill Jack sustained injuries in an automobile accident on 6/3/96. She was the belted driver of an automobile that was hit on the passenger's side by another vehicle. On 6/21/96, which is almost three weeks following the accident, Ms. Jack presented to the office of Dr. Adio for examination and treatment. Ms. Jack complained of neck pain radiating into the right arm and shoulder blade. The initial examination found decreased cervical spine flexion, positive cervical compression, positive Wright's, positive Adson's, diminished reflexes in the right upper extremity, and weakness of the right deltoid. The initial diagnosis included whiplash, nerve root irritation at C5/6, and thoracic outlet syndrome. The initial treatment plan was to consist of treatment three times a week that included spinal adjustment, ultrasound, traction, EMS, cold, myofascial release, and therapeutic exercises.

The progress notes from Dr. Adio's office showed approximately 46 dates of service from 6/21/96 through 10/17/96. The progress notes primarily contain the services rendered on each patient encounter with minimal subjective notations made. The treatment primarily consisted of passive therapy sometimes at the frequency of 6 units of passive therapy per date of service. I found only minimal notations of right medical knee pain or a lumbar spine complaint.

Page 2
Jill Jack

Ms. Jack underwent neurological evaluation on 8/1/96. The impression of this examination was "cervical radiculopathy, thoracic outlet syndrome, post traumatic headaches, and thoracic strain." Recommendations included a cervical spine MRI and an upper extremity EMG/NCV.

Upper extremity EMG/NCV revealed a right C6 radiculopathy. Cervical spine MRI showed spondylosis at C5/6 with no stenosis or nerve root compression. A lumbar spine MRI dated 8/6/96 revealed no disc herniations. Lumbar spine x-rays dated 7/16/96 showed minimal degenerative changes.

On 11/5/96 Ms. Jack presented to Dr. Sam Mixer for examination and treatment. The diagnosis included "acceleration/deceleration with resultant sprain/strain injuries and myofascial pain syndrome. C5 lateral disc protrusion with radiculitis. Thoracic outlet syndrome. Cervical, thoracic, and lumbar subluxation complexes." The initial treatment consisted of distraction, EMS, trigger point therapy, and exercises.

A reexamination on 12/6/96 found the patient 90% improved. The examination included only a cervical spine examination. Progress notes show 20 dates of service from 11/8/96 through and including 4/2/97, which is the last date of service provided for review.

Billings indicate that treatment rendered included office visits, myofascial release, therapeutic exercises, and neuromuscular reeducation. There were several consecutive dates where a comprehensive office visit was billed for.

PHONE CONSULTATION WITH THE ATTENDING DOCTOR:

On 4/16/97 I spoke with Dr. Mixer. He stated the last time he saw Ms. Jack was 4/11/97 and that treatment frequency is one visit every 3 to 4 weeks with discharge anticipated for one month. He states Ms. Jack had an exacerbation of her low back complaint. Dr. Mixer stated that the neck complaint is significantly improved.

CLINICAL OPINION:

I have been asked to address the reasonableness and medical necessity of treatment provided by Sam Mixer, D.C. to Jill Jack as a result of injuries sustained in an automobile accident on 6/3/96. I do agree with the application of chiropractic care to a degree in the management of this case.

Ms. Jack presented to Dr. Mixer on 11/5/96 for initial evaluation. The examination, distraction, and myofascial release would seem reasonable. The five dates of service from 11/15/96 through and including 12/2/96, consisting of a brief office visit, one unit of mechanical distraction, and one unit of myofascial release, would be considered reasonable.

The reexamination on 12/6/96, one unit of therapeutic exercise, and one unit on neuromuscular reeducation would be considered reasonable.

The treatment on 12/13/96, 12/15/96, 12/20/96, and 1/13/97 consisting of a brief office visit, one unit of therapeutic exercise, and one unit of neuromuscular reeducation would be considered medically necessary.

Page3
Jill Jack

Due to the fact that Ms. Jack did complain of ongoing cervical spine symptomatology when she presented to Dr. Mixer, it would be reasonable that she be given a
trial course of chiropractic care due to Dr. Mixer's treatment approach differing
from the first course of treatment. Dr. Mixer's treatment consisted of distraction
and an active care approach to treatment. There are 8 dates of service from
11/8/96 to 12/6/96. She was again treated on 12/13 and 12/20 of 1996 and was
not seen again until 1/13/97. Subsequent follow-up on 2/7/97 indicated that the
patient was doing well. Due to the minimum treatment required to resolve Ms.
Jack's symptoms and the gaps in treatment prior to 2/7/97 that Ms. Jack had
reached maximum improvement.

The records did indicate that she experienced an exacerbation of her low back pain
on 2/18/97. However, I do not feel that treatment for this exacerbation of low back
pain would be considered medically necessary as a result of injuries sustained on
6/3/96.

The first course of chiropractic treatment did not contain a diagnosis relating to
the lumbar spine. The only diagnosis with regards to the lumbar spine from Dr.
Mixer's office included "lumbar vertebral subluxation." The reevaluation on 12/6/96
did not contain an examination of the lumbar spine. The clinical impression or lack
of clinical impression to the lumbar spine fails to establish a basis for continuation of treatment beyond the 2/7/97 office visit.

CLOSURE:

The opinions rendered in this case are the opinions of the reviewer. This review
has been conducted without a medical examination of the individual reviewed. This
is based on documents provided to us by the provider with the assumption that the
diagnosis is true and correct. This report is a clinical assessment and opinion
conducted with the information available. It does not constitute per se recommendation for specific claims to be made or enforced.

Sincerely,

Gregg J. Fisher, D.C.
Licensed Chiropractor

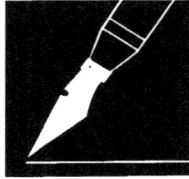

CHAPTER • TWENTY-SEVEN

FREQUENTLY ASKED QUESTIONS

1. I was conducting a phone consultation and the doctor continued to ask me questions about my practice—how many patients I see a week and how many reviews I have done. How do I handle this scenario?

   The purpose of the phone consultation is to give the doctor an opportunity to give verbal input regarding the case under review. This is no time to play "twenty questions." You would first ask the doctor to keep his comments to the case being reviewed. If he/she persists, ask again. If the interrogation continues indicate that you will terminate the phone call should the questioning continue. If you hang up, document the particulars of the conversation in the report.

2. What if the doctor tells me on the phone that he has a report he wants to fax to me?

   Under most circumstances you would never accept records directly from the provider. Ask the doctor to send or fax the records to the company who sent the file to you, the reviewer. The review company would then determine whether you will review the records prior to your final determination.

3. I was reviewing a case with a date of injury from 1989. I was asking the treating doctor about treatment and diagnostic tests prior to his beginning to see the patient in 1996. The treating doctor said that he did not need to do a complete history or examination because he is only a "referral provider." What should I do?

   Just because a chiropractor gets a referral from a medical doctor does not relieve him/her from taking a proper history and doing an adequate examination. The treating doctor must first establish the need for chiropractic care and this is done by history, examination, and reviewing ancillary diagnostic tests. As a reviewer, try to get as much information as possible, but if the treating doctor won't cooperate, you must base your conclusions on the available information.

4. The doctor under review requested a phone consultation but will not make himself available at a mutually convenient time. What should I do?

   You should make at least three reasonable attempts to contact the provider under review. You should attempt to hold the discussion at a mutually agreeable time. If the provider will not agree to a time, you should call his/her office at least three different days and ask if they will make themselves available. If they will not, document these attempts in your report and base your conclusions on the information available.

5. Where do I find work to do peer and utilization reviews?

   This depends on the state that you are in. In Pennsylvania, the Bureau of Workers' Compensation has a list of companies approved to do utilization reviews. Other states may be regulated by the insurance department. Regardless, you would find out which companies "broker" reviews and independent examinations and begin to market them. They would want to see your CV, sample reports, and a list of your charges. They would also want to be sure you had malpractice coverage for doing this type of work.

6. What should I do if I am sent a file to review on a good friend?

   If you are sent a file to review to which you cannot give an objective opinion, send it back. Remember, you are not an advocate for any of the parties involved. You are to give an impartial opinion of the case before you.

7. What should I do if I have doubt about a case?

   If you have doubt, treatment should be resolved in favor of the provider under review. This is written into the workers' compensation guidelines in Pennsylvania, but would apply whenever there is doubt on the part of the reviewer.

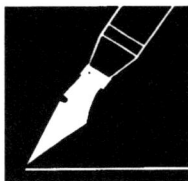

CHAPTER TWENTY-EIGHT

TEST YOUR KNOWLEDGE

This chapter is designed to see what you have learned from this material. If you don't know the answer to a question or want to review the material, you will be told where to go to find the answer. The chapter where the answer will be found is in parenthesis after the question.

1. What are the differences between active and passive care? (Chapter 1)

2. What are the components of a clinical impression? (Chapter 1)

3. Name two characteristics of a non-goal-oriented treatment program? (Chapter 1)

4. What are the criteria for supportive care? (Chapter 2)

5. What are the differences between supportive and maintenance care? (Chapter 2)

6. Explain the purpose of health care records. (Chapter 4)

7. Write an example of a treatment plan. (Chapter 4)

8. What are the eight parameters of the chief complaint? (Chapter 5)

9. What are the four delays to recovery found in the Mercy Guidelines? (Chapter 5)

10. Define SOAP. (Chapter 6)

11. Name five components of a reexamination. (Chapter 7)

12. Name three reasons why diagnostic procedures are necessary. (Chapter 11)

13. What are the five clinically necessary criteria? (Chapter 11)

14. What are the three phases of soft tissue repair. (Chapter 12)

15. Name at least four classes of adjunctive modalities. (Chapter 13)

16. Name at least four "red flags." (Chapter 16)

17. Name at least five procedures which are most likely to trigger a utilization review. (Chapter 17)

18. What are the six different areas to a peer review report? (Chapter 20)

19. What are the four components of a radiology report? (Chapter 21)

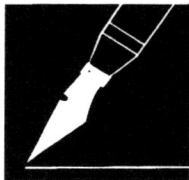

CHAPTER • TWENTY-NINE

PENNSYLVANIA LAWS

This chapter provides a brief overview of the peer and utilization review processes in Pennsylvania. Act 6 refers to the Pennsylvania auto law and Act 57 refers to the Pennsylvania Workers' Compensation Law. It is recommended that each person acquire a complete copy of each law. This chapter contains only excerpts of both laws.

ACT 57 (WORKERS' COMPENSATION) REVIEW PROCESS

INTRODUCTION

The utilization review process in the state of Pennsylvania is based on random assignment. A review is assigned at random to one of approximately 90 companies currently sanctioned by the Bureau of Workers' Compensation to administer the review process. Act 57 eliminated the reconsideration process that Act 44 provided. The next step following an initial determination is filing a Petition for Review of Utilization Review Determination to have a hearing in front of a Workers' Compensation Judge.

WHO CAN ASK FOR A UTILIZATION REVIEW?

An employer/insurer and the injured employee can file for a utilization review. Over 95% of all utilization review requests are filed by the employer/insurer.

WHAT ARE THE STEPS IN THE REVIEW PROCESS?

1. A utilization review is filed by an employer/insurer or the claimant. This request gets sent to the Bureau of Workers' Compensation.

2. The review gets assigned at random to a utilization review organization (URO). The URO has five (5) days to request records from the providers listed on the request form. Only those providers listed on the review request will be asked to send the records.

3. Providers have 30 days from the date of the request to mail the records to the UROs. Records are reimbursed at the rate of seven cents per page. The wording of the request letters is sometimes misleading. It is recommended that providers send all of the records for the work-related injury and not just

the records covering the treatment under review. Providers may also request to discuss the case with the reviewer prior to the reviewer's final determination.

4. The UROs assign the review to a doctor of same or similar specialty to complete the review. The URO has 30 days from the record deadline to do the review. (Total days to complete the review is 65 days from the date on the notice of assignment)

5. A face sheet package gets sent to all of the parties listed on the notice of assignment. This includes the face sheet, report, verification and petition for review form.

6. Each party has the option to file a petition for review of utilization review determination to have a hearing in front of the referee.

On 7/10/95 all UROs were instructed to not accept the following as records to review:

1. Do not accept summaries of medical records as documents to review.

2. Do not accept IME reports as part of the treatment records no matter who submits them.

3. Do not send Workers' Compensation Judges' decisions to reviewers as part of the records to review.

THE FOLLOWING AREAS OR ISSUES ARE NOT SUBJECT TO UTILIZATION REVIEW

• The casual relationship between the treatment under review and the employee's work-related injury.

• Whether the employee is still disabled.

• Whether MMI has been obtained.

• Whether the provider performed the treatment under review as a result of an unlawful self-referral.

• The reasonableness of the fees charged by the provider.

• The appropriateness of the diagnostic or procedural codes used by the provider for billing purposes.

• Reference to IME reports or opinions.

• The reviewers opinion on additional or alternative treatments or procedures which could have been administered.

• Other issues which do not relate to the reasonableness and necessity of treatment.

WHAT CAN BE REVIEWED?

All of a provider's treatment and referrals can be the subject of a utilization review. The referrals might be to another doctor, clinic, or for a diagnostic test. Section 127.470 indicates that reviewers can only determine the reasonableness and necessity of treatment.

SELECTED EXCERPTS FROM ACT 57

127.466 All reviewers must be licensed in the Commonwealth of Pennsylvania.

127.661 Each reviewer shall have an active practice spending at least 20 hours a week treating patients in a clinical setting.

127.467 Reviewers shall apply generally accepted treatment protocols as appropriate to the individual case before them.

127.469 The reviewer shall initiate discussion with the provider under review when such a discussion will assist the reviewer in reaching a determination.

127.470 Reviewers shall only decide whether treatment is reasonable or necessary for the medical condition of the employee.

127.471 Reviewers shall make a definite determination as to whether the treatment under review is reasonable and necessary. If the reviewer is unable to determine that the treatment under review is reasonable or necessary, the reviewer shall resolve the issue in favor of the provider under review.

WHAT ARE THE CONFLICTS OF INTEREST FOR UROs AND REVIEWERS?

1. Previous involvement with the patient or with the provider under review regarding the same underlying claim.
2. Performing precertification functions in the same matter.
3. Provided case management services in the same matter.
4. Provided vocational rehabilitation services in the same matter.
5. Having a contractual arrangement with any party subject to the review.

WHAT ARE COMMON MISTAKES BY PROVIDERS UNDER REVIEW

1. The doctor assumes that all of the records for additional providers will be requested. (Only those provided on the request form will have their records requested.)
2. The doctor does not supply documentation to fill gaps in treatment time. For example, the date of injury is 1989 and the patient presents for treatment in 1992. You need to show a clinical course to fill the gap in time.
3. No decrease in the frequency of treatment as the patient gets better.
4. Complicating factors are not found in the medical file.
5. Sending requested records to the insurance company or the Workers' Compensation Bureau.

WHAT ARE COMMON MISTAKES BY REVIEWERS?

1. The reviewer comments on treatment and dates of service that are not listed on the request form. Only the treatment and date(s) on the request form are subject to the utilization review.
2. The reviewer comments on one of the areas that is not subject to the utilization review.

ACT 6 (AUTOMOBILE REVIEW) PROCESS

INTRODUCTION

The automobile review process is based on the free market system. An insurance carrier contracts with one or more peer review organizations (PROs) directly. A PRO has the authority to evaluate the reasonableness and medical necessity of care, and the professional standards of performance including the appropriateness of the setting where the care is rendered, and the appropriateness of the delivery of the care rendered.

WHAT TRIGGERS A PEER REVIEW?

69.52(a) "A provider's bill shall be referred to a PRO only when circumstances or conditions relating to medical and rehabilitative services provided cause a PRUDENT PERSON, familiar with PRO procedures, standards, and practices, to believe it necessary that a PRO determine the reasonableness and necessity of care, the appropriateness of the setting where the care is rendered, and the appropriateness of the delivery of the care. An insurer shall notify a provider, in writing, when referring bills for PRO review at the time of the referral."

STEPS IN THE REVIEW PROCESS

1. A bill is referred to a PRO by an insurance carrier. The provider is notified.

2. PROs request records from the health care providers. The health care providers have 30 days to submit the records and billings. Bills, narratives and summaries can all be submitted for Act 6.

3. The initial determination is assigned to a doctor to review. The PRO has thirty (30) days to complete the review from the date the records were due. (The review may be tolled for twenty [20] days if additional information is required to complete the review.) The provider under review may request the opportunity to discuss the case with the reviewer prior to the reviewer's final determination.

4. Each party has thirty (30) days to submit additional records and request a reconsideration. (Remember loser pays.) The review can again be tolled in twenty (20) days if additional information is required to complete the review.

5. Reconsiderations must be done thirty (30) days from when additional information was received. Must be diplomat vs. diplomat for reconsiderations.

WHAT QUESTIONS ARE GENERALLY ASKED FOR ACT 6?

1. Determine the reasonableness and medical necessity of treatment rendered.

2. Has the patient reached maximum medical improvement?

3. Other questions may include determining medical necessity of diagnostic procedures, appropriateness of specialty referrals, durable medical goods, impairment ratings, etc. A peer review is necessary to deny payment for medical services. IMEs and other scare tactics cannot be used to deny payment!

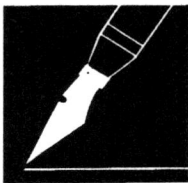

CHAPTER • THIRTY

TOP TEN LIST

This chapter is my attempt at a little humor.

THE TOP TEN REASONS DR. FISHER SHOULD APPROVE MY TREATMENT

10. I think I met you at a seminar once.
 9. I took one of your classes.
 8. I do peer reviews, too.
 7. I would give this treatment to you.
 6. I went to the same school as you did.
 5. My mother's name was Fisher.
 4. I just bought a brand new sportscar.
 3. The patient is one of the nicest patients I've ever had.
 2. Everyone says how good a reviewer you are.
 1. My kids are in college and I need to pay their tuition.

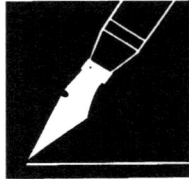

SUGGESTED READING

LITERATURE FOR DIAGNOSTIC ULTRASOUND

ACR Standards-Performing and Interpreting Diagnostic Ultrasound Examinations http://www.acr.org/standards.new/

Musculoskeletal Diagnostic Ultrasound: Non-Invasive Imaging is Here, *ACA Journal*, September 1995.

Ultasonic Measurement of Lumbar Canal Diameter: A Screening Tool for Low Back Disorders? *Southern Medical Journal*, Vol. 82, #8, August 1989.

Ultasound Diagnosis of Lumbar Disc Degeneration-Comparison with Computed Tomography/Discography, *Spine*, Vol. 16, #8, 1991.

Ultrasonic Level Diagnosis of Lumbar Disc Herniation, *Spine*, Vol. 15, #11, 1990

Facts and Fallacies of Diagnostic Ultrasond of the Adult Spine, *Dynamic Chiropractic*, Vol. 14, No. 9, 4/22/96.

LITERATURE FOR MUA

Chiropractors Rediscover an Old Way to Relieve Back Pain, *Your Health*, December 29, 1992.

Chronic Cervical Spine Pain Treated With Manipulation Under Anesthesia, *JNMS*, Vol. 4, #3, Fall 1996.

Manipulation Under Anesthesia of Lumbar Post-Laminectomy Syndrome in Patients with Epidural Fibrosis and Recurrent HNP, *ACA Journal* 1993.

Management of Cervical Disc Syndrome Utilizing Manipulation Under Anesthesia, *JMPT*, Vol. 16, #3, 1993.

Manipulation with the Patient Under Anesthesia, *JAOA*, Vol. 92, #9, Sept. 1992.

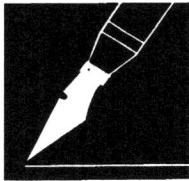

REFERENCES

American Medical Association. (1993). *Guides to the evaluation of permanent impairment*, 4th edition, AMA.

Barry, M. (1996). Facts and fallacies of diagnostic ultrasound of the adult spine, *Dynamic Chiropractic*, Vol. 14, No. 9, 4/22.

Bigos et al. (1986). Back injuries in industry: A retrospective study. Employee related factors. *Spine*, 11(3):252-256.

Bigos et al. (1994). *Acute low back problems in adults: Assessment and treatment.* U.S. Dept. of Health and Human Services Guideline 14.

Boden et al. (1990). Abnormal magnetic resonance scans of the lumbar spine in asymptomatic subjects, *J. of Bone and Joint Surgery*, Vol. 72-A, #3.

Capistrant, T., M.D. (1986). Thoracic outlet syndrome in cervical strain injury, *Minnesota Medicine*, Vol. 69, January.

Christiansen, K. D., D.C. (1991). *Chiropractic rehabilitation.* Vol. 1: Protocols, CRA.

Chusid, J. (1982). *Correlative neuroanatomy & functional neurology*, 19th edition, Lange Medical Publications.

Clinic Method II (1990). (Course Notes), Palmer College of Chiropractic.

Cox, J. M., Fromelt, K. A., and Shreiner, S. (1983). Chiropractic statistical survey of 100 consecutive low-back pain patients, *JMPT*.

Croft, A., Foreman, S. (1996). *Whiplash injuries: The acceleration/deceleration syndrome*, Williams and Wilkins.

Deans et al. (1987). *Neck sprain: a major cause of disability following car accidents, injury.*

Defranca, G., Levine, L. (1995). The T4 syndrome, *JMPT*, Vol. 18, #1.

Dorlands Medical Dictionary 27th edition. (1985). W. B. Saunders.

Downie, W. W., Leatham, P. A., and Rhind, V. M. et al. (1978). Studies with pain rating scales. *Ann. Rheum. Dis.* 37:378.

Dvorak, M., Panjabi, M., Novotny, J., Chang, D., and Grob, D. (1991). Clinical validation of functional flexion-extension roentgenograms of the lumbar spine, *Spine*, 16(8):943–950.

Evans, R. *Illustrated essentials in orthopedic physical assessment.*

Evans, Ronald, D.C. (1994). *Illustrated essentials for orthopedic physical assessment*, Mosby, 1994.

Fisher G., D.C. (1997). 36 Hour peer, Utilization Review and Independent Examination (Course Notes).

Fisher, G. (1997). "Becoming a Doctor of Documentation," Seminar by Progressive Seminars, Pennsylvania.

Fitz-Ritson. (1990). The chiropractic management of cervical trauma, *JMPT*.

Gatchel et al. (1995). The dominant role of psychological risk factors in the developement of chronic low back pain disability, *Spine*, Vol. 20, #24.

Gore et al. (1986). Roentgenographic findings of the cervical spine in asymptomatic people, *Spine*, Vol. 11, #6, 1986.

Haas, M., Nyiendo, J., Peterson, C., Thiel, H., Sellars, T., Cassidy, D., and Yong-Hing, K. (1990). Ineterrater reliability of roentgenographical evaluation of the lumbar spine in lateral bending, *JMPT*, 13(4):179–189..

Haldeman S., and Chapman-Smith D., M.D. (1993). *Guidelines for chiropractic quality assurance and practice parameters*, Gaithersburg, Aspen.

Hardy, M. (1989). Biology of scar formation, *Physical Therapy*, Vol. 69, #12.

Hohl. (1975). Soft tissue injuries of the neck, *Clinical Orthopedics and Related Research.*

Honsson et al. Findings and outcome in whiplash-type neck distortions, *Spine*, Vol. 19, #24.

Hooper, P. (1995). The ABCs of CTDs, LACC (Course Notes).

Hoppenfeld, S. (1977). *Orthopedic neurology*, Lippencott.

Huskisson, E. C. (1974). Measurement of pain. *Lancet* 2:127.

Jensen, M. P., Karoly, P., and Braver, S. (1986). The measurement of clinical pain intensity: A comparison of six methods. *Pain* 27:117.

Kawaguchi, Y., Tsuji, H., M.B. (1994). Back muscle injury after posterior lumbar spine surgery, *Spine*, Vol. 19, No. 22, pp 2590-2597.

Kellet, J. (1986). Acute soft tissue injuries: a review of the literature, medicine and science, *Sport and Exercise*, Vol. 18, #5.

Kormano. (1989). Imaging methods/lumbar spine, *Annals of Internal Medicine.*

Liebenson, C. (1996). *Rehabilitation of the spine: A practitioners manual.* Williams & Wilkins.

Magora. (1973). Investigation of the relationship of low back pain and occupation. *Scand J. Rehab. Med.,* 5:191-196.

Maurer. (1988). Biological effects of diagnostic x-rays exposure, *Amer. J. of Chiropractic Medicine.*

Murphy, Daniel, D.C. (1992). Whiplash and spinal trauma (Course Notes), Philadelphia.

National Academy of Manipulation Under Anesthesia Physicians Physicians Protocols and Standards, Atlanta, Oct. 26 and 27, 1996.

Ohio State Chiropractic Association. (1996). *Chiropractic treatment guidelines.*

Oklahoma Workers' Compensation low back guidelines, September 8, 1995.

Pennsylvania Blue Shield. (1997). *Procedure terminology manual.*

Petterson et al. (1995). Decreased width in the spinal canal in patients with chronic symptoms after whiplash injury, *Spine,* Vol. 20, #15.

Ransford, H. V., Cairns, D., and Mooney, V. (1976). The pain drawing as an aid to psychological evaluation of patients with low back pain. *Spine* 1:127.

Rehabilitation Guidelines for Chiropractic. (1992). CRA.

Sanderson et al. (1995). Compensation, work status, and disability in low back pain patients, *Spine,* Vol. 20, #5.

Simmons et al. (1995). Contemporary concepts in spine care: radiographic assessment for patients with low back pain, *Spine,* Vol. 20, #16.

Sinclair. (1988). Trends in radiation protection, *Health Physics,* 55:149-57.

Stonebrink, P.T. (1975). Guidelines for the chiropractic profession, *ACA Journal of Chiropractic,* June, Vol. 9, pp. 65-75.

Swartzman et al. (1996). The effect of litigation status on adjustment to whiplash injury, *Spine,* Vol.21, #1.

Terret, A. (1996). Vertebrobasilar stroke following manipulation, *NCMIC.*

Triano. (1991). *Standards of care: Manipulation procedures, conservative care of low back pain.* Williams and Wilkins.

Vernon, H. T., Mior, S. (1991). The neck disability index: A study of reliability and validity. *JMPT* 14:409.

Von Korff et al. (1993). Back pain in primary care, *Spine,* Vol. 18, #7, pp. 855-862.

Waddell, G., Main, C. J., and Morris, E. W. et al. (1982). Normality and reliability in clinical assessment of backache. *Br. Med. J.* 284:1519.

Wallis et al. (1996). Pain and psychological symptoms of australian patients with whiplash, *Spine*, Vol. 21, #7.

Williams, Glenn. (1986). Physiotherapy I, Palmer College (Course Notes), July.

Woolf, C. (1987). *Physiologic, inflammatory, and neuropathic pain, advances and technical standards in neurosurgery*, Woolf.